BY THE WATERS OF BABYLON

By the Waters of Babylon

One Family's Faith-Journey through Illness

Thomas J. Davis

WILLIAM B. EERDMANS PUBLISHING COMPANY
GRAND RAPIDS, MICHIGAN / CAMBRIDGE, U.K.

255 Jefferson Ave. S.E., Grand Rapids, Michigan 49503 /
P. O. Box 163, Cambridge CB3 9PU U.K.

Printed in the United States of America

00 99 98 97 96 95 7 6 5 4 3 2 1

Library of Congress Cataloging-in-Publication Data

Davis, Thomas J. (Thomas Jeffery), 1958-
By the waters of Babylon: one family's faith-journey through illness /
Thomas J. Davis.
p. cm.
ISBN 0-8028-4088-4 (pbk.: alk. paper)
1. Suffering — Religious aspects — Christianity. 2. Hope — Religious aspects — Christianity. 3. Lane, Melanie Ann. 4. Lymphoblastic leukemia — Patients — Family relationships. 5. Lymphoblastic leukemia — Patients — United States — Biography. I. Title.
BV4909.D38 1995
248.8'6'0922 — dc20 95-34279
CIP

Contents

Preface viii

PART I
THE EXILE

I. By the Waters of Babylon 3
II. Singers of Life, Not of Death 11
III. The Glassy Interval 20
IV. The Soul's Midwinter 27
V. The [F]Light of God 31
VI. The Little Children 38
VII. The Communion of the Saints 48
VIII. Walking in Darkness 56
IX. Rightful Minds 68
X. Holiday Hope 81
XI. To Sing Again (The Mystery of Living) 90

PART II
THE JOURNEY

XII. The Beginning 101

XIII. The Middle (Evil from the Hand of God) 113

XIV. The End 126

XV. Keeper of the Nail Clippings (The Sickness Unto Death) 142

XVI. The Lark Ascends 151

Epilogue: A Better Country 167

This book is dedicated to all the wonderful people who have been such a help to me: the Davis, Fodor, and Lane families; the members of that community of faith called the First Presbyterian Church of Danville, Indiana; colleagues; and friends in Danville, Indianapolis, and throughout the United States, with special mention for Kyle Pasewark. Special thanks also to Terry, Bob, Kelly, John, and Aaron. For all your kind words, helpful deeds, and concerned looks, I thank you. The fact that there is not enough room to mention all of you by name is witness to the abundance that characterizes God's mercy.

This book is a gift to my two dear children, Mave Lane Davis and Gwynne Lane Davis, whose smiles are the sunshine of my days and make glad my heart.

And, of course, this book is especially for Melanie, wife and dearest friend.

> "Lovely human eyes, yes —
> Green with swimming flakes of gold and brown.
> Yet mirrors of divine love."

Preface

This book is about faith, family, and illness. It is a reflection on the past few years of my life as I have lived it in relation to my wife's illness. It is about singing the Lord's song in a strange land; put another way, it is about having faith in God while traveling through an alien and hostile land — the land of a body ravaged. Though I was not the "sick" person in the family, the illness cast a long shadow over my life and the lives of my family. In these pages, by illuminating my own feelings along with those of my wife, my children, my family, and my church, I try to drive away the darkness. Or, if not to drive it away, at least to cast the shadow in stark enough relief to come to grips with the form of my fears and thereby give voice to my hope as well.

This writing represents my therapy. On these pages, I express feelings and thoughts I have trouble verbalizing to others. I am, I must admit, a misfit in today's psychotherapeutic culture. I am like Woody Boyd. Woody was a character on the popular sitcom *Cheers.* In describing his method for dealing with emotional problems to Dr. Frasier Crane, the show's psychiatrist, Woody once explained, "My feelings don't bother me.

I just keep cramming them down and cramming them down, further and further, so I don't have to deal with them." The good Dr. Crane, with a knowing glint in his eye, responded, "That explains a lot." And maybe it does with me, too. But what I have crammed down seems to have seeped out, to have gone from my fingers to a keyboard to a computer screen. Maybe Frasier would see that as a step in the right direction.

That said, I want to describe what this book is and what it is not. First of all, it is not a theodicy; I don't try to explain why bad things happen to good people. (That phrases the problem incorrectly, I think; theologically, I'm a Calvinist on this point. Experientially and emotionally, however, I'm not such a Calvinist, so that phrasing of the problem does carry certain emotional weight for me.) I do, of course, wrestle to an extent with that question (Why do bad things happen to good people?), but I give no systematic answer to it. Part of the point of this book is to deal frankly with the fact that the theodicy question is less important than other types of questions, at least on much of the journey through illness.

Second, this is not an "answer" book. I raise a lot of questions, explore them, and then leave them largely unanswered. A related point is that this book is not a systematic work of any sort. What I found throughout my wife's illness was that on some days one set of theological formulas helped me weather the storm, yet on other days I would find that same system sterile and oppressive, so I would turn to another source to help me cope with the theological issues at hand. Though I am intellectually a Calvinist at heart (saying it that way should reveal how I think Calvin's theology properly works), in this book I am sometimes wildly eclectic, espousing theories that in my purely intellectual moments I resist or reject. This points out the obvious — that religious life involves more than the intellect, and that a person who needs to wrench meaning from bad circumstance will often let emotional and spiritual needs override purely intellectual concerns. In other words, I drew strength from all the resources, intellectual and otherwise, that I had at my disposal to meet something other than a purely intellectual need. And this may also reflect the fact that, at the level of experience, good theology is less a system than it is a proclamation of something.

Finally, this book does not give a day-by-day account of the trials my family underwent — that would constitute frightful drudgery. But I have used a broad chronological framework — I start at the beginning of Melanie's diagnosis and follow things through to the present. Within that framework, I generally explore basic concerns that were present throughout Melanie's treatment process. I've also woven vignettes and reflections into the story.

What this book *is* is both hard and easy to define: it is my reflection on my wife's illness and how, through the resources of the Bible and Christian thought, I tried to understand how to be a Christian in such circumstances. I was aided in this process by friends and family, and by the wide communion of saints.

For anyone who has ever had to experience what my family has, I hope this book offers some consolation. Though it expresses my own feelings, fears, and hopes, perhaps what I have written will help give voice to your own.

PART I

THE EXILE

By the waters of Babylon,
there we sat down
and wept,
when we remembered Zion. . . .
For there our captors
required of us songs . . . saying,
"Sing us one of the songs of Zion!"
How shall we sing the Lord's song
in a [strange] land?

— Psalm 137:1, 3-4

CHAPTER I

By the Waters of Babylon

By the waters of Babylon,
there we sat down
and wept,
when we remembered Zion. . . .
For there our captors
required of us songs . . . saying,
"Sing us one of the songs of Zion!"
How shall we sing the Lord's song
in a [strange] land?

— Psalm 137:1, 3-4

I was sitting at my office desk on July 1, 1991, when the call came. My wife had gone to the doctor because of "lumps" on her head. There were no lumps there, really. I know. Several times she had asked me to feel along her head, to confirm for her what she felt — painful knots, aching bumps that hurt so much she couldn't sleep at night. But there were no lumps.

It was summertime, and the immediate future looked

bright. We lived in a neighborhood and a house that we really liked. We had two beautiful children: Mave, who was five, and Gwynne, who was two. Melanie was closing in on the final quarter of her first year at her new position as pastor of a Presbyterian church in rural Indiana. I was growing into my job at a nearby university, where I teach the history of Christianity and serve as managing editor for a scholarly journal. I had finished my dissertation, and so I was looking forward to receiving my Ph.D. After years of struggle and sacrifice during an eternity of schooling for both Melanie and me, our family seemed to be getting on its feet in a substantial way. Except for the lumps.

The lumps themselves were just one of many symptoms Melanie had experienced during several months of strange and undiagnosable pains. Two months before, Melanie had gone to the emergency room of the local hospital because she thought she was having a heart attack. The doctors did an EKG and blood work — she was fine, they said. They gave her some ibuprofen to take for what they thought might be a pulled muscle in her chest. A few weeks later, she had gone back to a doctor — this time because her leg hurt, particularly around the knee. She had begun to take it easy, to stay off the leg, and take the ibuprofen. The doctor had seemed skeptical. She saw that Melanie had been in a few weeks earlier and basically dismissed her complaints. She did not examine Melanie, just told her to keep resting the leg. Another prescription for ibuprofen was doled out, and Melanie was sent on her way. But her leg still hurt.

I was thinking about all this as I sat at the desk in my office. Truthfully, I had been slightly annoyed at times over the past couple of months. For one thing, I had had to do more of the housework because Melanie hadn't felt well enough to bother with it. And the doctors hadn't seemed to think anything was really wrong. And now the lumps.

Well, not just the lumps. Some people thought Melanie

"looked bad." Melanie and I had just come back from a long vacation to Georgia, where our families lived, and many of the folks who saw Melanie for the first time in many months thought she looked pale; her mother was especially worried. And I suppose she did, though sometimes it's hard to notice gradual changes in a person you live with every day. Lumps and looks sent her to the doctor — lumps because they hurt Melanie, and looks because Melanie's mother called every night to ask when she was going to get to a doctor. So Melanie finally went to the clinic again.

When Melanie called, she was near tears. Her blood counts, compared with those taken just six weeks earlier, were terrible. Her hemoglobin was half what it had been; her white blood cells and platelets were worse yet. The doctor had told her it might be leukemia. It might be leukemia. It could be leukemia. More tests would tell. Tomorrow.

I made my way out the office door with a manuscript in hand: typeset pages for Indiana University Press that had to be delivered that day. So I decided to leave work (it was early afternoon), go to Bloomington to drop off the pages, and then go home. On my way out, someone called after me. My fumbling response was, without further explanation, "Melanie may be real sick." It sounded funny. Real sick. I should have said "really sick," I suppose. But either way it wouldn't have sounded right. Melanie was healthy. Melanie was strong. How could she be really sick (or real sick)? The words sounded false, tin-cup syllables clanging in the wind. It was not true. And so I went to Bloomington.

I thought about more than lumps and looks as I made my way down Highway 37. Real sick. Very sick. Serious illness. I tried a variety of labels, but none of them seemed to stick. I grasped for some concept, some idea, for comfort — for the right words to distance me emotionally from the words that suddenly melted away in my mind, to be replaced by an image from my days in Chicago. The first few times I rode the elevated train from Rogers Park to Hyde Park, I noticed what seemed to be a nice green park, but it was surrounded by concrete walls. On subsequent rides, when I paid better attention, I realized it was not a park but a cemetery. I looked at the walls. Spray-painted in ugly red were the words "If you can't beat 'em, join 'em." I had tried to clutch onto something to help me understand and master what was happening; now, something clenched its ephemeral hands around my mind — this image of fear. If you can't beat 'em, join 'em. Death. People died of leukemia. People died. They filled graveyards with concrete walls, walls desecrated by smart-ass kids who think they're immortal. And, of course, it happened — I saw a tombstone with Melanie's name on it. It was a vision that came after me as I rode down the highway, alone, and I was afraid. The sun went behind a cloud, I think. The world seemed dimmer.

I delivered my pages, my mind beaten with dark thoughts. But things seemed to brighten up once I finally got home. I ran up the stairs, crossed the front porch in a couple of steps, and went inside. I held Melanie, and the news no longer seemed as bleak. She had talked to the oncologist, who had informed her that the internist she had seen could well be mistaken; there were several explanations for low blood counts. Don't panic. Wait until we know something for sure. That seemed to be the best course, an optimistic course.

Mave and Gwynne had their annual physical checkups scheduled for the next day; the date had been set months ago. After some discussion, Melanie and I decided that I should take the kids to the pediatrician — no use having to reschedule — and she would ask one of her church members to take her to the oncologist. It was the sane thing, the rational thing to do. We kept reassuring each other. There's no need to panic. There's been no real diagnosis. It could just be a virus, the oncologist had said. We went to bed and slept the agitated sleep of uncertain hopes and fears.

The children's trip to the doctor went as usual. Mave and Gwynne were fine. I began to discuss with the pediatrician the fact that the children's mother might have some sort of virus — her blood counts were down pretty low. Yes, there was an outside chance of leukemia, but the oncologist had said (perhaps I should have said "we had heard" — *oncologist* sounded serious) that a virus of some sort or anemia probably best explained her blood tests. So we wanted to arrange for a blood test for the children, just in case Melanie did have this virus. (No, I asked for the test because Melanie *did* have a virus, I was sure.) We wanted to make sure that the kids hadn't picked it up, too. Then the children and I went home, singing songs, as we often did in the car.

I expected Melanie to be home when we arrived, but she wasn't there. Of course, I reassured myself, you can spend all day at the doctor's office when you're perfectly healthy. I imagined additional blood tests were needed to pinpoint the virus. And so I waited.

I was looking out the window when Melanie and Betty, who had taken Melanie to the doctor, drove up. I ran out the door to find out how everything had gone. Tears welled up in Melanie's eyes. Betty handed me her car keys and said she would watch the kids while Melanie and I went over to her house to talk. I think Betty may have hugged me as she handed me the keys; I'm pretty sure she hugged Melanie. My mind was filled with the image of the graveyard again — If you can't beat 'em, join 'em. I wanted to reach out to Melanie, but it seemed instead that something reached out for me, and it was something that frightened me.

We talked for about an hour at Betty's house. Melanie had been diagnosed with acute lymphoblastic leukemia. She told me everything she could remember about what the doctor had said. A bone-marrow test had verified the presence of leukemic cells. This was an aggressive disease, he had said. Very aggressive — without treatment, she would be dead in a matter of weeks. Aggressive diseases call for aggressive treatments. He had told her to be at the hospital at 7:00 a.m. the next day for admission.

While still at Betty's, I called my department chair and told him that I wouldn't be at work the next day, and that I didn't know when I would be in again. Then I said, for the first of many times, "Melanie has acute lymphoblastic leukemia." It was hard to say; the words sounded funny in my mouth. Acoot limfoblastic lookeemeah. The syllables were slurred; I mumbled a bit. I still have trouble pronouncing the words. Sometimes I stumble and have to repeat a part of the phrase twice to get it out. And then I was asked, again for the first of many times, "Is there anything I can do?" The question confused me, because I didn't know what needed to be done. It was like asking a lost man for directions; I was the lost man in unknown territory. "No" sounded tinny and ungracious, but it was the only answer I could come up with. No. No, not right now. Maybe you cannot help ever. I was wandering along in a strange land with no signposts.

That night we prepared for the hospital. One of the things we had to do was shop for new nightgowns and underwear for Melanie. We told Mave and Gwynne that there was something wrong with Mommy's blood and that she had to go to the hospital to get it fixed. Mave, our five-year-old, said, "But you can't live without blood." Yet her somber analysis almost immediately gave way to joy — she enjoyed shopping, and she picked out some colorful underwear for Mommy. With the shopping done and the children informed as best Melanie and I knew how to do it, we settled in for the night.

I then did one of the dumbest things I've ever done in my life. I went to my study and picked up the *Reader's Digest Great*

Encyclopedic Dictionary, a hefty tome. Someone had given it to us as a gift fifteen years ago, when Melanie and I were first married. I almost never used it, but I knew it had a medical dictionary, so I took it to our bedroom and plopped down on the bed beside Melanie. My fingers nervously thumbed to the medical dictionary, and I soon found the entry headed "Leukemia." I began reading out loud to Melanie. There was lots of information about blood cells and abnormal growth; there was also the last line that read "This disease is always fatal." Since I had been skimming ahead while reading aloud, I faltered. Melanie asked me what was wrong. "Nothing," I said. "It's just that this thing says a lot more about blood cells and stuff. I think we better wait to see the doctor and let him explain more fully what it all means." We went to sleep, such as it was, Melanie with vague anxieties about what tomorrow might bring, me with much more sharply defined fears about death.

For the first time I realized how much I had taken Melanie's life for granted. Of course, all married couples take each other for granted to various degrees. We had been lucky because, as we had done so, we had still been enough in love to recognize it and try to combat that malaise of marriage which deadens one's senses to the joys of life together. Nevertheless, we had had our dry spells, just like everyone else. Now I felt guilty. It's one thing to take one's marriage for granted; now I realized that I had very much taken Melanie's life for granted. Maybe this is normal, but it didn't feel normal. So I tumbled through sleep with a sense of sinfulness — the sins of omission are as grievous as the sins of commission, as all prayerbooks remind us. For the first time, the language did more than settle into my theological conscience as doctrinally correct — it hurt. And I was sorry.

When morning finally came, we were up and ready. Betty came by to stay with the kids, and Melanie said good-bye to them. Mave looked up after Melanie told her she loved her and said, "Mommy, I don't want you to go." Melanie cried; tears welled up in my eyes; the children cried. Melanie didn't want to go, either, and I certainly didn't want her to go. Yet she and I were already well along a path that was taking us where we didn't want to go, and the trip to the hospital was just the barest physical symbol of a journey into a Babylon of physical, emotional, and spiritual boundaries that would seek to hold us in exile. I had once written a poem for my wife, comparing our marriage to a song. The last line read, "We are the music, and you are my love." I wondered now, as we were being carried along the route of exile, whether our music would ring true to what we both had always believed and professed. How could we sing the Lord's song in this strange land? And did we even want to try? Would the memories of our personal Zion, the Zion of a relatively easy relationship with God untested by the fires of stringent adversity, carry our tune along, or would cacophony result? Time would tell.

CHAPTER II

Singers of Life, Not of Death

Be singers of life, not of death.

— From a sermon I once heard

I took over Melanie's pulpit for her. The doctor had said that she would be in the hospital for a month or so; after that, she would still need a lot of help and wouldn't be able to return right away to her preaching duties. So, since I am also an ordained Presbyterian minister, I took over for her.

I had preached for Melanie before, but the first time I did so after she was hospitalized was eerie. I stood in her pulpit, wondering how long it would be hers. I looked out over the congregation; by this time next year, would some of them be dead? My mother-in-law sat near the front, off to my right, trying to maintain her composure. Would my sermon help?

Melanie and I had decided one thing: to remain upbeat and positive. At least, that's what Melanie wanted — from herself and others. She didn't want people with hang-dog looks moping about; she forbade phone calls of the weeping-and-wailing sort. She wanted to concentrate on getting well; she didn't want negative images or feelings. She especially didn't want to hear "Poor thing, how can I help you?" — which, she was afraid, would lead the one offering consolation to break down and degenerate into sobbing "Oh, I'm sorry, so sorry." Melanie had to focus on her self, on her recovery; she didn't have time to make others feel better about her illness.

What she did want to offer, however, was an affirmation of life, of the goodness of life. And, to that end, I was to be her voice in the pulpit — not a voice that bemoaned the fact of sickness and death, but one that sang the glories and possibilities of life. This is, after all, the basic Christian belief, once you peel away all doctrine: life is good because God makes it; to trust God is to trust life's goodness, even in bad times. As Christians, then, we are to be singers of life, not of death. The resurrection is about the wrenching of life from death, and whether one takes the story literally or allegorically or poetically, the meaning plays out the same: life is good enough that God bothers sustaining it; God sustains us. Paul put it another way, but I think he meant the same thing: in life and in death, God saves his children.

There were people in the congregation that morning who had not heard that Melanie was ill. So I had to announce the fact. It was the most difficult part of the service for me. How do you announce something of this sort to people who care deeply about their minister? I ran through several variations in my mind. One seemed too formal and cold; another seemed sappy and overly emotional. There was no room for humor, something I normally rely on too heavily to ease my way through sticky, uncomfortable, or tricky situations. (Finally I even axed from consideration the line "As you can tell, I'm not Melanie" — banal, but always good at eliciting a chuckle of pity.) I came out with a simple, straightforward announcement.

"Many of you already know this, but for those of you who don't, Melanie was diagnosed with acute lymphoblastic leukemia (acoot limfoblastic lookeemeah — I had so much trouble pronouncing it) on Tuesday. She was admitted to the hospital on Wednesday, where she'll undergo chemotherapy for about the next month. I'll be filling in for her in her absence, and I'll keep all of you abreast of her condition."

Visible shock and audible gasps rippled through the congregation. A few people cried. But in the spirit of singing life from the pulpit that morning, I immediately went on, leaving little time for folks to settle into their fears, fears for Melanie and fears for themselves, though that would surely come. Instead, I read a letter from Melanie to the congregation, a practice I would continue for as long as Melanie was in the hospital. On that first Sunday morning of her absence, this is what she had to say to her people:

> Dear friends:
>
> I have often said that life is an adventure. Sometimes it seems we take some very unexpected turns. This particular turn in my life is not, however, a dead end. I want to get well; I want to live. I have a lot of sermons yet to preach before I even make a mark on Billy Graham's record. I am aware that this unexpected turn comes at a difficult time. You and I are still in that getting-to-know-you year. There are lots of ideas percolating in my head about where we could be going over the next several years. It is rather a frustration not to be able to act now on some of those things.
>
> What I ask from you is that we rally together. I need to know that as a community you are gathering for prayer and worship to remember me and the many others in our group who need to be lifted up to God.
>
> Life in our community needs to keep going. Please don't put things on hold because the preacher's got cancer. I will be back soon. Don't hesitate to call me or ask Tom about anything. Grace and peace to you all.
>
> *Love, Melanie*

The great thing was that the congregation did exactly what Melanie asked in that first letter. They gathered for prayer, they worshiped, they remembered her. That support would be crucial during the next several months. And it was very real.

The service continued. I had thought carefully about what to preach that morning. I decided it would be a mistake to try to preach as if it were a normal Sunday morning, unrelated to the fact of the preacher's cancer. So I turned to Job and read various passages. This is what I had to say, hoping to call a strong tune to life's song:

> The ironies of life can sometimes overwhelm us. There are two ironies that come to my mind this morning as I look back on the past week.
>
> Just one week ago today, Melanie stood here and preached a sermon on God's care for the sick and dying. Remember Jairus, a daddy grabbing at Jesus' arm — "Please, master, come heal my daughter." That's the image Melanie started her sermon with. And here today, in collective prayer, we grab for God's arm — Please, Father, come heal our minister; wife; mother; daughter.
>
> One week ago today, I handed a completed bulletin to Sam Thompson at White Lick Church. My sermon title? "Why Do Bad Things Happen to Good People?" And this morning I stand before you with that very question on my lips — except now it is not a rhetorical question for a catchy sermon title, one that I hoped people would tie into and recognize from Rabbi Kushner's popular book. It's the question that could frame my entire existence, if I let it. What a difference a week makes. A sermon on healing, a question about God's goodness, and a diagnosis of leukemia. It's an irony that breaks hearts.
>
> The first thing to admit is that, in the face of any devastating news or events, we look up to God and ask "Why?"

Why is this happening? In the book of Job, the good man Job needles God for an answer. More than that, he cries out that any just judge would be on his side. Job screams for an umpire to weigh his complaint against God. Why, God? Job called out. Why me?

It was not because Job had done evil. The Scriptures are plain — Job was a good man. He did not in any sense deserve his suffering. And that is good for all of us to keep in mind.

Of course, sometimes it's hard to believe that. As we drove to the hospital on Wednesday, Melanie looked over and said to me, "I know better than to think this way — my theological training and pastoral care training tell me this is not the right way to think. But I gotta know," she said. Then she looked hard at me. "Do you think I've done something to deserve this?"

I slowed down, took her hand, and said, "Melanie, you're the best person I know. You don't deserve this. Your own sermon last week said that loud and clear. God doesn't work that way." Yet, as you can see, in times of deep trouble, we all ask, Why me?

I think what we have to remember is that there's a mystery to life we cannot penetrate. We simply don't know why bad things happen to good people, and, frankly, the Bible really doesn't even try to tell us. Maybe that's because what it does tell us is something more important, and something more sustaining — that God is with us, and loves us, and will take care of us in all of life's circumstances. Now, this doesn't take away the sorrow or sadness. Remember, even Jesus wept when he heard that his friend Lazarus had died. Saying that God cares for us doesn't take away the pain, or the hurt, or the anger that comes up in circumstances that devastate people. But to say we trust God's promise that he loves us and cares for us is to say that when the pain and hurt, anger and sorrow, have settled into the depths of our breaking hearts, they find there a peace and comfort, a courage and trust, that recognize that in life and in death, in health and in sickness, God saves his children. For it is in him that we live and move and have our being. What we are is his, and he'll take care of us.

This is another way of saying that in times such as these, God doesn't give answers, but gives himself. That's what Job eventually learned. And it's something Jesus tried to teach us when he instituted the Lord's Supper: "This is my body," he says, "my very self, broken for you." And when he says "Take and eat," he's saying that as much as bread becomes part of us when we eat it, so Christ becomes part of us when we trust in him. In times of trouble, God is not far away, but near. Next to us. In us. Nourishing, strengthening, feeding our souls unto eternal life. In all of life's circumstances, God loves us, cares for us, and gives himself to us. I believe that. Melanie believes it. And, I hope, so do you. Because if we do believe the Gospel, we can affirm the words of that great old hymn:

> In heavenly love abiding,
>   no change my heart shall fear.
> And safe is such confiding,
>   for nothing changes here.
> The storm may roar without me,
>   my heart may low be laid.
> But God is round about me,
>   and can I be dismayed?

May it be so for us. Amen.

The service ended. I talked to a lot of folks about Melanie — her condition, her prospects, and her treatment. They expressed genuine concern and care, both for Melanie and for us, the family. I don't know if the sermon helped anyone else sort through the situation, but it did lay out for me the principles I would try to abide by in dealing with what would come to seem like a daily disaster. But now that the principles were like so many cards laid out on the table, the question became, Was I bluffing or holding aces? What I wished someone would and would not ask me, and thus the question I had to deal with on my own in silence and solitude rather than in community, was this: Did I believe what I said in the sermon? For me, the single prospect of the entire service that was both the most frightening and the most exciting was the one that entailed a courageous parishioner coming up to me afterward and saying, "Nice sermon, Tom. Do you believe it?"

I still wrestle with that question. If I'm a singer of life, is the song true? Am I moved enough by the words and melody of Christian faith to accept them, believe them, sing along with them? Am I, after all and when all is said and done, a singer of life, or someone who sits in the audience, swept away by the beauty of the music, but an observer nonetheless? Are the words, is the Word, true enough to believe?

Martin Luther was once asked if he believed the Gospel as strongly as he preached it. In a remarkably honest response, he said, "No, and I don't believe the Apostle Paul believed as strongly as he wrote, either." Some may take this answer to represent a lack of faith; I do not. Instead, Luther seems to be pointing to the fact that maybe good news, the Good News, has a life and power of its own separate from the messenger. To use more strictly theological language, the Word and those who deliver the Word are instruments of grace, means appointed by God to announce life in the midst of a dead and dying world. The message is God's: it is true; the messengers are God's also, in the sense of belonging to him. And, hopefully, the truthfulness of the message makes the messenger, the vessel, true — true in the sense that he or she is attuned to the message. But one should also realize that the message is so big, so powerful, so Good, Absolutely Good, that the messenger cannot contain the message. In this sense, neither Luther nor Paul nor I can believe in a great enough way to do the message justice; it is more than we are. But it is precisely because it is more than we are that it can uphold us, in spite of our weak belief, and sometimes in spite of our disbelief.

The Psalmist says, "My soul melts away for sorrow; strengthen me according to thy word" (119:28). Here is what I look for in God's Word, and in my words: strength to affirm life. I am sad; I cannot squeeze belief out of the resources of a melted soul. I am formless and runny, like melting ice. Do I believe what I preach? No. I cannot. But I can listen to God's Word, preach God's Word, and pray that it breathes over the waters of my soul to order faith out of the chaos of unbelief. God, give me your Word; God, give me a song — this is my own prayer.

A fellow named John Nevin once remarked that Christianity is not so much a doctrine or a moral system as it is a life. All our Christian doctrines and all our Christian ethics serve to illuminate that life. I like that. To be a Christian is to live a life with Christ, through Christ, in Christ. To be a Christian is to be part of a living body, a living fellowship, called Christ's body. In it we give our lives and are given life, true life, immortal life. Christianity is life together.

If that's so, then maybe Melanie's parishioners were right in not asking me if I believed what I preached; maybe it's just us minister types, especially academic types, who are so hung up on belief, how it is defined, the rules for thinking rightly about Christianity. For us the question becomes not "Do I believe what I preach?" but "Do I somehow or another live what I preach?" Not in the sense of some strict legalism; no one lives the Gospel in the sense of fulfilling its demands. Rather, it is a question about whether or not I live and act and strive as though the Gospel is true. Is my life strung so as to sound truth in my comings and goings?

If we talk about Christianity in this way, I think the "Do you believe" question takes a back seat to hope. Matters of belief may or may not spur action; may or may not give comfort; may or may not matter in any real sense. Lots of people, as both Martin Luther and John Calvin remind us, believe the facts about Jesus' life, death, and resurrection without that affecting one bit how they live their lives. But if one lives in hope, that's a different situation altogether. Hope looks forward, acts, moves, as if the best good news of all is, in fact, the best good news of all because it is so. Hope motivates. Hope is an attitude. Most of all, if I live my life in Christian hope, the best good news of all is the best good news of all because it is good news for me personally. To live in Christian hope may involve believing correctly, but it is not limited by that narrow way.

Hopeful people sing. In sixteenth-century France, followers of John Calvin sang the Psalms as they were carted off to the stake. They sang joyfully as they were burned. Finally, their executioners began to cut out their tongues before they were killed in order to silence their songs of hope. Singing life in the midst of death, even without tongues, these folks were filled with a hopeful melody. Within them burned a fierce joy that wasn't tamed even by the prospect of death.

As I shared my wife's tribulations, my fervent wish was to have this kind of hope for both of us. I hoped I could sing.

CHAPTER III

The Glassy Interval

Let him lean
Against his life, that glassy interval
'Twixt us and nothing: and upon the ground
Of his own slippery breath, draw hueless dreams,
and gaze on frost-work hopes. Uncourteous Death
knuckles the pane, and —

— Thomas Lovell Beddoes, 1803-1849

I began to live my days with images of living and dying. Or, at least, I tried. The snapshot pictures in my brain were mostly of dying, despite my best efforts to see life. Sometimes I wondered if I was sane, or if I was simply evil; surely a good person would imagine good things. But most of the time I didn't.

Melanie's images, at least the ones she told me about, were about living. In the beginning, there were those brief exchanges in which she would say to me, with childlike honesty, "I don't want to die." But those brief moments were caged in the first few days of her initial hospital stay. After that, she didn't speak of dying — though of course in a way she did; it was simply couched in terms of the alternative. A strongly expressed wish to live carries with it an implicit desire not to die. But the images she shared with me were about living.

The clearest memory I have of her mental portraits of the future comes from one afternoon in the fall, after Melanie had come home from her first stay in the hospital. We were in the living room: I was sitting on the sofa, she in the rocking chair. We were just passing time (although "just" doesn't really apply when talking about time) when she seemed to get very sad. I asked her to tell me what she was thinking about. As tears began to run down her cheeks, she said, "I'm thinking about rocking on our front porch in our retirement years. Just being together." Melanie wanted life so badly, and so she thought of a pleasant time in the future, one that bespoke a happy and satisfying past, a future time that implied a past. Yet her tears reminded both of us that it might not be so. The image, though, was hopeful.

How unlike my images. It wasn't just that I couldn't imagine life; my fantasies swirled like dark clouds until the image of a funeral emerged, and I was sucked down the funnel to sit and watch the death rites of my wife. The things I saw were crystal clear, too real, and very scary. I was confronted with details: I surveyed the faces of all the people at the service; I listened to the words of the minister; I led the procession after the funeral; I made the trip to the graveyard; I participated in the graveside service. All these events played out before me like scenes from a movie. And they disturbed me.

What was most disturbing was that I thought I actually knew what that all meant — that I was preparing for Melanie's death, not her life. Was she about to step through that glassy interval; was her life as fragile as that? I pondered the words Davies quoted. Some of them jumped out at me, causing me to reflect on the contingency of life.

The most compelling phrase was "frost-work hopes." Is life itself nothing more than a frost-work hope that gives the appearance of substance and, especially, beauty, but that melts under pressure or the harsh light of reality? I was reminded of when I was a child, six or seven. On cold winter mornings the frost would form on my bedroom window. What beautiful shapes. Crystalline images ran over the glass, casting reflections of design and connectedness that delighted me. But, of course, two things were fatal for these frosty masterpieces. If I touched the glass, the thin-layered ice immediately melted. And if the sun came up or out from behind clouds, the light would more slowly, but just as surely, erase the work of the nighttime frost artist. If I reached out to touch my wife, really touch her, would whatever it was that made her *her* melt before me? And if I tried simply to think through what was going on, apply canons of reason to this insane situation, would the comeliness of her existence melt before the heat, leaving me with a rational, albeit lonely, assessment of the situation? Was I gazing on a frost-work hope?

Well, of course I was, in a sense. All bodies die. The human race has a one hundred percent mortality rate. Samuel Johnson called it the incessant mortality of the human race. We all die; we're just not very good at dealing with that fact. Most of the time we are insulated from death — by our health-care system, by our hospitals and nursing homes, by our middle-class existence that sees death as an unseemly interruption of the natural flow of things. People may die young in the Middle East, or in Africa, or in war-torn sections of Northern Ireland. But in America, we like to tell ourselves, that doesn't happen. For most of us, death is never very close until it is too close.

Medieval folks lived much more closely with death, partly because squalor and disease and primitive medical practices made death commonplace. In many ways, death became an obsession; books proliferated on the art of dying well. One particularly popular theme in the artwork from the latter part of the Middle Ages was the dance of death. In most of these pictures, bodies in various states of decay were shown dancing on graves. Yet these skeletal phantoms retained enough of their clothing that they could be identified as peasant, clergy, or lord; physical size indicated whether they were young or old. All people die, in all states of life. The dance of life always gives way to the last dance; finitude promenades. The frosty ball thaws away to nothing.

Still, knowing about finitude is not the same thing as knowing finitude. I can rationally explain (and preach) that all things come to an end. It's natural; all things finally cease. Life in general is a glassy interval that's like Alice's looking glass: at some point, you slip through it. Life in particular — that's another matter. It's not so comforting to know that all things end when the person you love may end. The uncertain nature of life may make for a good, general sermon illustration; but the uncertain nature of *Melanie's* life did not bear too much relation to sermon writing. Her contingency was both painfully real and yet anesthetically unreal, and neither the reality nor the unreality fit neatly into a sermon outline.

As I thought about finitude and death and the knowledge of them both, I kept remembering an embarrassing event from my younger days. As a teenager, I had been a "preacher" in the Baptist church I attended. Looking back on it, and now being very different religiously, I see it as a bad thing to let a young man (a boy, really) do. But there I was, "licensed" to preach at the age of fifteen. And preach I did, based on absolutely no knowledge of anything important. I exuded the odious certainty of the ignorant. The embarrassing event that continues to surface in my mind has to do with my Grandmother Burda's death.

I knew little about her death — just that it had been somehow or other unpleasant. It wasn't until my mother came to help out with Melanie that I asked specifically what had killed her. Total renal failure, my mother told me. My grandmother had died in pain. Since she had been unable to process her body's waste fluids, her body — her legs especially — had become bloated with waste, which excreted from her pores. As a teenager I had heard that Burda had prayed to God to let her die. I now better understood why. I also understood how one could pray in this situation; perhaps it is because one believes God is good and will answer prayer. But deeper than that, I think, is a prayer that comes from someone who believes — no, feels — something more primal about God: that God is powerful. Burda had prayed not to a good God but to the primevally puissant God who held the key to her release from torment.

I remember the day of her funeral. I was being my preacherly self in the only way, perhaps, a teenager in that role can be — I was acting smug and self-assured. I can see it all so clearly. It was morning, and the sun was out. My sister passed me in the living room as we were getting ready for our trip to the church. I felt the need to pontificate. "Everyone shouldn't be so sad," I said. "Burdie's in heaven with God now. If we're Christian, we know that. We should be happy she's with God."

Imagine one person saying that to another. Of course, you probably can — it's been said many times. It's a coping device of sorts, and an altogether bad one. If I wanted to deal with my grandmother's death that way, I suppose that was my decision. But to try to convince someone else of its truthfulness borders on the demonic.

I've read more of the Bible now than I had back then — read it in the sense of paying attention to it. One of the few times that Jesus cried was when his friend Lazarus died. Sadness at someone's death, even from a biblical perspective, is appropriate. I think what those confused lines about being happy that a loved one is dead are meant to convey is the sense of hope that, at some level, runs beneath the currents of our laments. Yet, how crudely expressed. I wince when I think back on my grandmother's death and my essentially unfeeling chatter primarily because I now have a much greater appreciation for why it is that Jesus wept. That glassy interval is a bone-chilling reminder of the nothingness that threatens all our hopes and dreams, feelings and loves, creations and imaginations.

Of course, the problem is compounded by the fact that death itself doesn't have to actually come in order to kill us. The prospect of death is enough, when it is close enough, to start the process by killing off what is good and hopeful and joyous in our psychological and spiritual lives. And my mental life was filled with images of Melanie's death.

What was being strangled was my imagination. I simply couldn't imagine life in five or ten or twenty-five years with Melanie by my side. My anti-imagination was at work — anti-imagination that can see no further than the worst possible outcome; anti-imagination so brimming with the fact of illness that it spilled over into pictures of death. My dreams, if such poor constructs could indeed be referred to by that noble appellation, were indeed hueless; my mind was haunted by gray nightmares. No — better — gray daymares; the colors of my days had all run dry.

Other images came to me, particularly from the Psalms. I didn't know whether to be comforted by them or to run as fast as I could from them. They seemed so apt in their description of my spiritual state, yet I was so afraid to accept the words of comfort. Their depiction of my experience was striking — existentially, I was the Psalmist in distress: "For day and night your hand was heavy on me; my strength was dried up as by the heat of summer" (32:4). Was this experience God's hand on me? Was I being punished for sin? I felt dirty — a man of poor imagination who could not think of God's power to heal or help. Was that a sin? It might be. If it was, from whence would my consolation come?

One thing I had so much trouble with was the Psalmist's notion that it is God who breaks so he can heal, if called upon. Once-tidy Bible verses broke against my mind like giant, wild ocean waves about to overwash my sanity. "Therefore let everyone who is godly offer prayer to thee," the Psalmist advises. If one does so, the Psalmist guarantees, "at a time of distress, in the rush of great waters, they shall not reach him" (32:6). Yet the one who saves, at least according to the Psalmist (and my own religious tradition), was the one who had hurt me. "Let the bones which thou hast broken rejoice," the Psalmist cries (51:8). Why? Because the sacrifice acceptable to God is a broken spirit, a broken and contrite heart. Does God break the spirit so he may console it? The Psalmist indicates that God will not turn his back on such a spirit. Maybe we must be broken before we understand how it is in God that we live and move and have our being. I was broken but not consoled.

Of course, the problem was with me. With my bleak imagination, I simply couldn't imagine praying to God at that point in time. So I remained alone in the face of that glassy interval. And if I felt that way, how lonesome Melanie must have been.

CHAPTER IV

The Soul's Midwinter

In the bleak midwinter,
frosty wind made moan.
Earth stood hard as iron,
water like a stone.
Snow had fallen, snow on snow,
snow on snow.
In the bleak midwinter,
long ago.

— Christina Rossetti, c. 1872

I never knew I could be so tired. Although I tried to keep my chin up (literally), the burdens of life weighed me down. Melanie needed me, and the kids needed me. I didn't want to be a bear to live with, so I tried to be as cheerful and understanding as possible, living out a lie that I hoped gave my family strength. But I was dying the slow death of a tired person; how long could I continue?

Yes, when I listed the things I had to do, it sounded like

a lot, but should I feel so overwhelmed? I continued to teach and work as the managing editor of a scholarly journal; I did the cooking, cleaning, and washing; I was responsible for the children — Melanie was home, but she was often too weak to deal with them very much at all. In addition, I tried to help Melanie out, and that involved at the least taking her to her many doctors' appointments as well as administering the chemotherapy (as much as possible) at home so she didn't have to spend so much time in the hospital; I also filled in for Melanie at her church, preaching every Sunday, and I taught Sunday school. Most importantly, I think I provided the psychological stability for my family and, to a lesser extent, for the church. I think that was the most tiring thing. A cheerful, optimistic face in the face of darkness. My smile was what was causing my soul's distress. I had no one to talk to; I didn't confide in others about how hard my situation was. When people finally got around to asking how I was, I gave them a bromidic, buck-me-up "I'm fine. Doing OK." But I wasn't fine. The moaning winds of despair frosted my mind; I could smile because the moisture in my lips had frozen hard as stone; and my heart was so heavy that it felt like it must be iron. I was trapped in a bleak midwinter.

I scared myself with my thoughts. One way to rest would be to die. I imagined my own funeral — there he is, dead of a heart attack, probably. I would hover above the casket, just like in the TV shows that deal so pathetically with death, listening to the sadness in people's voices as they said, "Wasn't he a swell guy?" I heard them talk about my fighting the good fight, how I had carried a burden heavier than anyone should have to carry alone. Of course, it had all been too much. Finally, I would come to my senses, realizing that, in the afterlife, God probably doesn't let us engage in such blatant and egotistical self-pity. Still, the image remained.

But when I wasn't engaged in such self-pity, I found myself

thinking the unthinkable. I was tired, so what were my options? I could never leave; I wouldn't want to. I was too proud to send out a real plea for help, to have someone come and stay and take care of me while I took care of Melanie. How would I rest? The solution, at moments, was terrifyingly clear: I would drive myself into a tree. I thought about it, riding down the road. Not in a schizophrenic way — there were no voices. But there were photographically clear images. I would drive into a tree and I would live. But I would be so badly hurt that I would have to go to the hospital for an extended period of time. And while I was in the hospital I could rest without shame. Fell asleep at the wheel, I'd say — exhaustion, pure and simple. Then maybe everyone would know how tired I was.

Of course, no one knew, not even Melanie. I didn't tell her, refrained from complaining, because I didn't want to add to her already considerable burden. If I was tired, how must she feel? There were times when she had practically no white blood cells; her hemoglobin was sometimes only half of what it should have been. Yet, she didn't share her tiredness with me; I knew she didn't want to burden me with her complaints, either. Out of our love for one another, we each held back, trying to be considerate of the already overloaded psyche of the other. But sometimes, in our concern and care for one another, I wonder if we weren't knocking out from under each other the only support we had. Sometimes I think what we did was like kicking the arches out from under a wall so that it wouldn't be burdened by the weight. Of course, it's that countervailing weight that holds the wall up; without the weight of the arches, the wall falls.

At my most exhausted, there were other, even darker thoughts I harbored. Things that, even now as I look back, I cannot bring myself to write down for fear that someone will judge me too harshly without understanding the extreme stress I was experiencing; I also don't write about such things because of the people who could, even now, be hurt by them. There are those who depend on me who cannot now be, and perhaps never can be, strong enough emotionally to hear my thoughts and understand; I fear the repercussions that revelations of this sort can bring. Suffice it to say that my dark thoughts filled me with self-loathing — and here, I think, is the self turned in on itself, seeking only to fulfill its own desires. If Martin Luther was correct in saying that sin is being curved in on ourselves, I was the greatest of sinners. I looked only inward.

I was beginning to feel like some sort of loathsome monster. What truly loving husband and father could wish such a thing as I was — or, if not wish for it, at least entertain it in his imagination? It was around this time, while I was cleaning the house, that I picked up one of the notebooks that Melanie wrote in. When I glanced through it, I realized she was having the same thoughts as I was. Yet she recognized them for what they were — expressions of terrible anger at the unjustness of it all. After honestly expressing herself on the page, she turned around and wrote this prayer: "Dear God, this is my anger. Take it from me."

In the honest expression of her thoughts, words she wrote only for herself, she reached me, and I was helped. Because then I realized how much we needed each other, how much we both needed support. I wasn't alone in my dark imaginings; here was one I loved who was having many of the same grim feelings and thoughts I was enduring. And even though I never mentioned to Melanie that I had read her words, after that I felt we were closer, bound together in adversity not only to look at the dark side of life but to confront our own dark natures. And as I trod the paths through the shadowed confines of my soul's midwinter, I felt heartened. Not because the atmosphere was less bleak, but because I did not have to walk through it alone.

CHAPTER V

The [F]Light of God

"I'm sick! I can't be closed up in this thing.
Get me out! . . . Jesus."
"Jesus been a long time gone."

— dialogue from
Flannery O'Connor's *Wise Blood*

"Lo! I am with you always,
to the close of the age."
— Matthew 28:20

Mark Twain once said that faith is believing what you know ain't so. In a rather insightful way, Frederick Buechner has pointed out what it is that lends credence to Twain's assertion for so many people: of all missing persons, God is the most missing. Many books have sought to answer the "Why" of suffering. Why do I have to suffer? Why does a good God, if all-powerful, allow people to suffer (or, put more strongly, inflict the suffering)? Yet the real crisis for the sick person and those who suffer along with her or him is not "Why, God?" but rather "Where, God?" Where are you?

Still, I sometimes act as if the Why question is important. I'm not sure it is. Certainly, as an intellectual question, it can be stimulating. But as applied to life? I'm not so sure.

In one of my classes, "Introduction to Religion," we spend a class period or so on the Why question. Of course, in the syllabus, I use the ten-dollar word — theodicy. Theodicies are ways to try to explain that God is both all-good and all-powerful in light of the evil and suffering in the world. After Melanie got sick physically and both of us were suffering mentally and spiritually, I stood up one day to talk to my class that fall semester about theodicy. It gave me an unreal feeling.

First, I presented the problem: If God is good, he can't be all-powerful, or else there wouldn't be so much suffering in the world. What good person would want that for another? So, if God is good, he must be limited in some way. Of course, the reverse of the argument is this: that if God is all-powerful, he must not be good. That is the sadistic view of God.

Then I laid out the various explanations that have been used throughout Christian history to try to get at this problem. And as I ran through each argument and each counterargument, I thought that it missed the point altogether to speak in this way. Still, I continued to try to impress upon my students the importance of learning these concepts. Somehow, I think the dull glaze over their eyes simply mirrored the glaze over my own mind.

Of course, the most obvious response to the problem of suffering — and one that people who are not suffering have, historically, been all too quick to seize upon as an explanation — is that people suffer in order to pay for their sins. In my reading of the sixteenth century, every time an enemy suffers or dies, it is proclaimed God's just punishment. Here is a response that has taken the notion of divine justice, scaled it down to human terms of the big payback, and then pawned it off as God's will.

On this particular day, as I tried to rationalize for the class how this interpretation of the world and its problems could be justified, referring to no less an authority than Saint Augustine to give it a whiff of tradition and respectability, a song kept running through my mind. Back when I was a kid, there was a Southern gospel group that, as only a Southern gospel group could, would blare out the words "God's gonna git ya for that, God's gonna git ya for that. Ain't no place to run and hide, 'cause he knows where you're at." Had Melanie been "gitten" by God? I didn't think so. But I'm sure some people might have offered a different opinion, because they would see that as the only way to protect God's goodness.

The second traditional theodicy asserts that suffering is a trial of faith, a burning fire by which the soul is purified as it sojourns through life. This seems to be found in the book of Job: Job is an innocent man whose faith is tested by God to show the Tempter that Job is righteous. Job passes the test in the sense that he does not curse God. I like Job, but not because he passes the test. I like Job because he stands up to God and demands justice from him. Rather than curse God, Job confronts him. Of course, Job will back down after God starts the predictable "I am God and I can do as I like and who are you to question me." Yet, for me, the important part is the engagement with God on a level that's human, honest, angry. That is faith — not the banal affirmation in the face of adversity.

Still, the trial-of-faith explanation seems pretty ungodly of God, too. Run-of-the-mill finitude mixed in with the rigors of life in general seems to present enough of a trial without a heaping serving of additional suffering dolloped on top. So, though I droned on to my class, I didn't pay much attention.

Then there's the final explanation — that suffering is a

teacher. According to this argument, the person who has suffered learns things about herself and about life she wouldn't have known otherwise. This argument has some real possibilities, not so much for really serving theodicy's purpose — to get God off the hook — but for wrenching meaning and something good out of a bad situation. Of course, this argument can be distilled into the fatuous caption for Iggy posters — "Sometimes things go wrong so you'll know when things go right." I think that when things go wrong in a really big way, it so overwhelms a person that there's no real possibility of contemplating the "rightness" of life; but it does open up opportunities to see the goodness in life.

In some cases, like my family's, suffering does teach love. But not in every case; I can imagine that there are people who suffer in isolation; they have no one to turn to, and no one turns to them, only away. But people turned to us. Even though I didn't ask for help often enough and often felt overburdened, we did get frequent assistance. Family and church friends helped keep things going in our house. Church friends kept the kids when Melanie and I needed that, and occasionally they surprised us with meals so that I didn't have to cook. Family members, all of whom live several hundred miles away, came regularly and provided a type of weekend relief so that I didn't have to constantly keep up with the kids and household chores; it gave me some time to relax. People prayed for us — people we knew and people we didn't know. Melanie and our family were on church prayer lists from Massachusetts to Minnesota to Georgia. I saw love during Melanie's illness, and so did she. If, as the poet A. R. Ammons says, our world is such that "it can't get loose from / meanings and the mind / can't pull free of it," then love expressed is one of the meanings that came out of my family's suffering, though I know it all too often doesn't for others. No grand theodicy here, just an individual's instinct for survival; order imagined is better than chaos.

There are other things that suffering teaches — empathy for others who suffer, for example, and patience. Yet I believe those things pale beside the big question: Is the suffering offset in any way by these lessons? Or, in my family's case, wasn't there a better way to learn love? Or is love always — maybe only — revealed in suffering?

As I kept talking, my own questions and my class's questions all blurred together. No, academically styled theodicy wasn't much help for me, and I doubt it helped the class much, either. They stared; they wrote down what I said. Later they would regurgitate it, and then they would be free of the food for thought I was trying to ram down their throats. It was junk food, anyway.

Of course, I think that sometimes I try to intellectualize meaning too much. Maybe meaning is not so much something served up on the platter of the intellect as it is an understanding shared among souls, an understanding that is not spoken but felt. An understanding that leans on The One Who Understands for support. In other words, meaning may be more an understanding relationship than a mental syllogism. "Why, God?" is replaced by "Where, God?" because the need to be with Understanding, rather than to possess understanding, underlies the quest for meaning.

So, where is God amid the suffering? I wasn't asking that as a big question — Where is God in the world's suffering, in the hunger, the wars, and so on? Although this question is important, the "Where" at this point was personal, just as my family's suffering was personal. I sought a presence. Though church and family might serve as God's hands and feet, ministering to me, what I wanted, what I needed, was more: an overpowering sense of presence that I could float in, be swept up in. Individual acts of love weren't enough — I wanted an ocean, with an ocean's swell. Sometimes I think I felt it; most often, I just wished I did.

I have never considered myself a mystical person. I was raised a Baptist and am now a Presbyterian minister with a strong affinity for John Calvin's theology. That characterization doesn't logically lend itself to mysticism. I am skeptical of mysticism's claims and of the mentality; to my mind, it has often seemed like a running away from the intellect. I find myself siding with Calvin in terms of thinking that what's important in Christianity is the *knowing*. My attitude is reflected in the way I like to refer to a group of mystics; just as you have a herd of cattle or a gam of whales, when you have more than one mystic, it's a muddle — a muddle of mystics.

Yet, despite this attitude of mine, I found in this time of crisis that knowing didn't amount to much; a presence was what I needed. And maybe even John Calvin knew that; after all, when it's all said and done, what one is supposed to know so well when one is done with the knowing is that there is a mystical union between Christ and his people. That's not stressed as often as it should be when Calvin is taught. What I wanted was a union of presences.

Of course, what would that be like? Would it come in the ocean swell I wanted? Or is the presence of God most often felt in God's absence? Does overwhelming absence clue us in to a real presence of God in our lives? This seems like nonsense; at the very least, it seems paradoxical. But that's one of the things I became more comfortable with: paradox. Life is messy and unsystematic; should faith be any different? In my life I hold contradictory opinions, work at odds against myself. Maybe a living faith shares those attributes — which would also explain why every theology that tries simply through clever academic sleight of hand to systematize faith, make it neat with no wrinkles, fails. Professional theology, which usually stakes so much on the intellect and the systematic ordering of knowledge, may have so little impact in the churches for exactly this reason: it presents a permanent-press faith, one that looks neat on the surface but that cannot possibly survive the wrinkly vicissitudes that our existence imposes on us.

Given my greater tolerance for paradox, I became less impatient with the more nonsensical-sounding writings of someone like Luther, who knew a good deal about God's presences and absences. What he wrote may sound like nonsense, but some of his phrases rang so true for me that I thought my head might crack open. One in particular comforted me — not because I could understand it, much less explain it, but because it mirrored what little apprehension I had of God. Luther talks about "the wonderful memory and visitation of God, who is most mindful when he forgets and visits most when he abandons." Rather paradoxical, but Luther explains the meaning of this phrase, as he does everything important he has to say, in relation to the cross of Jesus. We all too often forget the cross; but it is here, in the central event of the Christian story, that we have confirmation of Luther's insight. We forget that the whole Christian schema of salvation is centered on a moment in time when God seems to have forgotten and abandoned Jesus. "My God, my God, why have you forsaken me?" Jesus cried out. Yet here also, the absence bespeaks presence, as the writer of the Christian story knew.

Psalm 22, which cries the same cry as Jesus and speaks of total abandonment, cries that cry nonetheless to the God who is not there; the final affirmation of both the Psalmist and Jesus the Risen One is that God is there even in the absence. God most filled the world when he abandoned Jesus on the cross. Absence assures us of presence; you don't miss what was never there to begin with. It turns out that the most marvelous light of God, his illuminating, swelling, filling presence in our world, is figured for us in the way that we miss him. Absence becomes presence; darkness becomes light. Jesus has been a long time gone while all the time he's been very near. The flight of God and the light of God are the same.

CHAPTER VI

The Little Children

Let the children come to me, and do not hinder them;
for to such belongs the kingdom of God.

— Luke 18:16

Jesus loves the little children,
all the children of the world.
Red and yellow, black and white,
they are precious in his sight.
Jesus loves the little children of the world.

— Author unknown

See what love the Father has given us,
that we should be called children of God;
and we are!

— from the baptismal service in
the Presbyterian *Worshipbook*

The Little Children

The day before Melanie was to go to the hospital, we sat down with our older daughter, Mave, to explain to her what was going on. We told her, in what we considered to be five-year-old terms, what was wrong with Melanie. "Mommy has to go to the hospital so they can fix her blood." We told her about the illness and how long Melanie would be in the hospital. After we had finished, Mave looked up and said simply, "But you can't live without blood." That's true, we answered, but the hospital would make everything better. Still, Mave had given voice to our fears, and her own.

When Melanie and I left the next morning, the good-byes were tearful, of course. Even Gwynne, our two-year-old, cried. She couldn't understand what was going on or why, but she did know that the most important person in her life was leaving, and she sensed from the rest of us that it wasn't a normal leaving. Normally, when a mommy leaves, there's no question she'll come back. On this morning, there was, and that was plenty of reason to cry.

Melanie and I knew a few things about children: that they are remarkably resilient little beings, but that they also feel the same things adults do but don't express them in quite the same way. My resolve was to try to remember both, to try to hold both together. Just because they would be sad, which they would be, didn't mean it was the end of the world, I told myself. Don't make things worse by either dwelling on the bad or trying to "make it go away"; give them a chance to come to terms with it on their own. Just because they might seem happy and normal, don't make things worse by trying to lacquer normality over the situation in an attempt to preserve a false sense of happiness; be in tune with their unspoken or subtly expressed emotions that will surely seep out around the edges of their lives, whether during playtime or dinnertime or any other time.

I needed to listen to them, and I did. So I heard Mave

and Gwynne playing dolls and talking about the mommy dying and the children having to fend for themselves. I had to care for these children, and Melanie had to care for them too, in the best way that she could.

Melanie was creative; she began to write bedtime stories for Mave and Gwynne from her hospital bed in order to fill the hours and to maintain her sense of connectedness with the girls. They didn't come to the hospital every day because it was a fifty-mile round trip; I tried to drive them in every other day. And when we were there, the visits were short because the girls quickly tired Melanie, especially the longer she was in the hospital. So Mave and Gwynne didn't have much physical contact with their mom for four weeks or so. Yet she was with them in those stories she wrote, stories that I read to them. Saint Bernard of Clairvaux once said that the soul is present more where it loves than where it lives. That means love rather than space is the real criterion for meaningful presence — the idea of the presence of love has always been the real impetus, I believe, in every attempt to understand the Eucharist in terms of a real presence of Christ. If Bernard was right, then Melanie's soul was present to the children through her love, mediated through my reading her stories to them. They felt comforted and safe — "mommified," for lack of a better word — when I read those stories.

Some of the stories were about when the children were born. Other stories were more of a mix of fantasy and reality, a blending of the severe reality we were facing with the gladness of hope. One in particular served as almost a visionary experience for me, helping me to see hope — not just feel it but actually see it. Although the story was written for Mave, it had — and still has — the character of an epiphany for me in its beautifully crafted recognition of life as it is combined with a desire for life as it might be. I choked back tears the first time I lay beside Mave in her bed and read it:

The Little Children

There once was a little girl named Mave. She had a Mommy and a Daddy, a sister named Gwynne, and a cat named Waifer. Just as it was time for Mave to get a new puppy for her birthday, her Mommy got very sick and had to go to the hospital. It had been a long, hard week for everyone.

One night, Mave's Daddy took her up to bed. They read a book and listened to the tape of Mommy singing Mave's favorite bedtime songs. Then Daddy kissed Mave goodnight and left the room.

Just as Mave was closing her eyes, she saw a tiny purple star land in her room near the bed. The purple star turned out to be a little fairy, and up close it looked more like a flower than a star — it was a purple flower fairy. She told Mave she had come to give her special fairy wings. Mave jumped out of bed and ran to her window. Suddenly, the window opened, and Mave had purple wings on her back and shoulders. The little fairy said, "These wings are very special — they will take you to see your Mommy." Mave was soon flying through the air. She could look down and see the lights and cars traveling along the road.

After a little bit, Mave saw a big building. It was the hospital where her Mommy was staying. In one room, Mave could see another beautiful purple light. The light was Mommy, shining with a set of wings on her shoulders and back, too. Mommy told Mave that the fairy said they could go to the zoo together.

As they walked through the zoo, they stopped to watch the tigers play a late-night game of jumping into the water after a ball. Next, they decided to go over to the farm section. Mave and her Mommy climbed over the fence and went into the goat barn. There were several new baby goats, and they played with them. Then they fed the goats some hay.

Then Mave and her Mommy went over to the carousel.

Mommy turned it on, and each of them took turns riding all the different animals. After many rides, Mave sat with her Mommy on a nearby bench and snuggled up close to her, listening to the snores of sleeping animals and watching the stars.

Suddenly, Mave began to feel her pillow against her face in the sleepy darkness. Mommy was tucking her back into bed. She kissed Mave goodnight and said, "I love you." Mave fell sound asleep.

The next morning, Mave sat up in bed and wondered if it had all been a dream. She checked under her nightgown — there weren't any wings. Then, on her shelf, Mave saw something sparkle. It was a tiny purple flower. Mave knew then that it had not been just a dream. She put the flower in a special place and went down to breakfast to tell Daddy about her adventure. She hoped that the good fairy would come again soon. And she could hardly wait to call Mommy!

I, too, hoped the good fairy would come again soon, bringing good news.

It was hard, in its own way, for Mave and Gwynne to go to the hospital to see their mother. First of all, it was, for them, an interminably long trip — twenty-five miles. So, by the time we got there, they would usually be pretty high-strung from having been cooped up in the car. But sometimes they would be asleep — Gwynne was especially prone to nap on the way. And waking up a child from a hard sleep to carry her into a hospital where she had to be relatively quiet and fairly calm wasn't always easy.

At first the girls were fascinated by various aspects of the hospital itself, so they concentrated more on the surroundings than they did on their mother. Even though I understood why this would and should be the case with small children, understanding didn't always help. During those first few visits, I found myself getting very angry with the kids for not paying enough attention to Melanie. Of course, they were paying attention in their own way, but I wanted them to be more grown-up about things — which meant masking their feelings and doing what they ought to do rather than what they felt like doing. Both "sides" frequently became exasperated: their behavior frustrated me, and mine frustrated them.

Three things they loved. The first was the hospital gift shop, where I always treated them to candy — often as a bribe, I must admit. All different kinds of goodies, lined up at a child's eye level. Somewhere out there is a monster who sucks the patience out of adults, and he spends most of his time designing displays so that they are most attractive to young children. I grew to hate that monster.

Mave and Gwynne also loved Melanie's hospital bed because they could move it up and down with the touch of a button. At first Melanie indulged them. She liked being moved up and down, and she enjoyed the girls' delight in the wonders of the bed. But as Melanie grew weaker, as her treatment made her sicker, she had less and less energy, and less and less patience, for bed play. Then it became a constant struggle to keep the kids' hands off the bed button once Melanie had had enough. Several visits were ruined — or at least on the edge of ruination — because of that button. I ended up wishing the girls had never found out about it; they seemed more interested in making Mommy go up and down than in making Mommy feel loved. Of course, I was applying adult standards to them; but, because of the circumstances, I often tried to squash the child out of them. I wanted them to behave and express themselves like adults; I wasn't much fun for them.

The third thing that Mave and Gwynne loved were the surgical gloves that became standard accessories in the room. Melanie was soon put in protective isolation; since the chemotherapy was killing off her white blood cells, she had to be protected from all germs — including ours. So the kids and I had to put on gloves and masks and gowns when we entered the room. To help the kids adjust to this process, one of the nurses showed them that the thin rubber gloves could be blown up like balloons — made into huge, bloated hands with five fat little fingers. You could do two things with the glove/balloon: tie the end, or let the air out so that the glove flew around the room. It was a nice gesture; the nurse was trying to help entertain Mave and Gwynne. Of course, just like the bed, the gloves became the focal point of visits. And so, like the bed button, the glove balloons had to be vetoed.

What Melanie and I discovered was that the visits actually went better if we did one of two things. The first was to let Mave, our five-year-old, visit Melanie without her two-year-old sister. By herself, Mave was calm enough to sit up in bed with Melanie while Melanie read her a book or just held her. These were very good visits; mother and daughter and dad all received something they needed — an expression of love. Then Gwynne could come in for her special time with Mommy — usually after a satisfying trip to the gift shop. And then she would curl up next to Melanie, glad for the comfort of her Mommy's touch.

The other thing we began to do, when Melanie felt well enough, was to meet out in the lounge. Melanie would don mask and gloves and gown, grab her IV pole, and roll down to an area that overlooked the front entrance. There was plenty of space for the kids to run around in, and there were two TVs. Here, in a more appropriate space with enough room for the kids to let off steam, visits were much more pleasant. They were longer visits, and although Mave and Gwynne spent a fair amount of time satisfying their childhood curiosity about any number of things, they also spent time with Mom.

Having a sick mother is hard for small children. Even

when Melanie was discharged from the hospital, things were hard — perhaps harder than they had been when she was in the hospital. When Melanie was there, she was removed from the home environment, in a special place to make her better. It was hard for the kids not to have their Mom around, but at the same time they found it comforting that the atmosphere at home didn't change too much while Melanie was confined to a hospital room. But once Melanie came home, Mave and Gwynne both had to make a very difficult adjustment. Mommy was home, but things were not the same.

Melanie was still, of course, very sick. Her intensive chemotherapy had weakened her considerably, and so she wasn't able to come home and assume her normal role; in fact, she wasn't able to do that for almost the entire length of the treatment process, which lasted about ten months. She slept a lot. And when she wasn't asleep, she was resting. We had to put Mave and Gwynne in day care for three days a week (Mave was in kindergarten, but the class lasted only a few hours a day); I stayed home the other two days and tried to work at home. So Mommy was home, but she wasn't. Kids who were used to having immediate and constant access to Mom were now denied that comfort. And I often served as the buffer between Mom and daughters. There was nothing harder than having to sit at the bottom of the stairs that led up to the bedroom and serve as a physical barrier to children who wanted to be near their Mommy. Mave and Gwynne expressed their frustration with anguished cries and tears, sometimes beating me with their little fists. I think they began to feel excluded by Melanie's withdrawal — something necessary for Melanie if she were to heal, but exasperating and painful for them, because I think they interpreted it as rejection.

Even when Melanie spent time with Mave and Gwynne, she was very tentative with them at first. Melanie was fragile, and she knew it, though it was hard to convey that to the girls.

When she was in the hospital, she had had a catheter put into her chest so that she could have blood drawn and chemo drugs injected. The catheter needed daily care: cleaning and flushing — and it represented a lifeline to Melanie. Especially at first, Melanie feared that Mave or Gwynne might jerk on the tube, pulling it out or, at the least, hurting her. And she didn't want to be hurt any more than she had been already. So, even while she held the girls, she often laid a protective hand on her chest, a visible reminder of her fear and fragility. Life with mother was not — simply could not be — the same.

The girls adjusted, but it was difficult for them. They wished for the mother who was well.

The Wednesday before Thanksgiving, I took the girls out for a hamburger. I was exhausted. Melanie had been home for three-and-a-half months, but the day before, she had been admitted to the hospital again; after a chemo treatment she had gone downhill very quickly, much too fast. When she had gone to see her oncologist, she was very ill: she had a fever of 103 degrees, her heart rate was nearly 150, her blood pressure was 80 over 60, and the roof of her mouth was covered with sores. He immediately sent her to the hospital.

The night before, one of the elders of the church had died. Since Melanie was sick, I had filled in for her at the funeral. Although another minister presided — Melanie felt so ill that she knew she couldn't handle the service — I participated, reading Scripture and praying at the graveside. Images of death — Melanie's death — overtook me. I was psychologically overtaxed; everywhere I looked, I imagined I saw people attending Melanie's funeral.

To top it all off, I was supposed to preach at the community Thanksgiving service that night. So there I sat, burger in hand, nothing in mind, and rather aimlessly asked Mave what she was thankful for in her life. A normal Thanksgiving-type question. I asked it primarily to occupy her so I could rest before trying to put together a sermon in the hour between mealtime and church time. She rattled off the usual list — she was thankful for food, her friends, school, her toys. For as much as I was listening, she might as well have been saying, "Blah blah blah, blah blah blah." Then she said something unexpected, and, thankfully, I heard it: "I'm thankful that I can ask God to make my Mommy better." Here was a child expressing thankfulness that there was a God she could ask for important things.

Two things happened then. First, I realized I now had my sermon. There was enough in that sentence to unpack for a lifetime. Second, I realized that I hadn't really asked God to make Melanie better. Oh, there had been prayer time in church and prayer time at night with the girls, but I had had no prayer time of my own. In my busyness, I had forgotten to pray the most important prayer I could pray: Dear God, make Melanie better. My five-year-old daughter had reminded me of my privilege and my responsibility: to treat God as a real figure, and to expect God to act and respond.

As a child of God, I had the right to ask, but I had not. In nearly five long months — from July 3 until the end of November — I had not asked God for anything. After that, I did. Thank goodness I had a child to remind me how to act as a child of God. In all of her attempts to deal with having a seriously ill mother, Mave remembered to pray. No wonder Jesus said that we must become as children to enter the kingdom of heaven.

CHAPTER VII

The Communion of the Saints

I looked, and behold, a great multitude
which no man could number, from every nation,
from all tribes and peoples and tongues,
standing before the throne and before the Lamb,
clothed in white robes,
with palm branches in their hands,
and crying out with a loud voice,
"Salvation belongs to our God who sits upon the throne,
and to the Lamb!"

— Revelation 7:9-10

Revelation speaks in beautifully poetic language about the community of saints: many people, of all different sorts, white-robed and circled around the Christ figure. I like this image of the communion of saints because I think it is, poetically, more powerful than Paul's somewhat labored description of the church as the body of Christ, though that image, in its way, is also helpful. But the white-robed chorus, joined in their differences by a common cry of salvation before our Lamb, is better for me. I like the notion of white-robed saints in a circle — it's more egalitarian than Paul's notion of members (though Paul, in his clumsy manner, is trying to move in that direction). The image of the lamb also appeals to me more than that of the head of the body. The latter is cerebral and controlling, which, in the proper context, is an appropriate image of Christ. But the former reminds us that what brings together white-robed saints from all nations is a victim, one sacrificed, who has suffered and borne sorrow. This is the Christ whom a sick person and her family needs; and it is the palm-waving chanters who cheer the suffering ones.

And it was cheer we needed, and cheer we got. While in this lifetime no saint is pure, God blesses the charitable act so that it at least is able to reveal the type of blinding purity of love he carries for us. We are blessed that he does so through us.

The community of saints rallied around our family in a variety of ways. All of them were helpful; some were inspiring. The cards they sent were especially heartening. Melanie received numerous cards, full of good wishes and prayers. At first there was a trickle, but as the word got out about her illness, the trickle became a flood. While Melanie was in the hospital, we began to build a wall of cards so that she could constantly look at a visible expression of the saints' concern. I began at the top of one wall, and I worked down. Once I got below bed level, where Melanie couldn't see the cards very well, I began working on the adjoining wall. Some of the cards were quite serious and "Christian"; others were humorous. Some were expensive store-bought cards; others were homemade. Some people sent more than one card. One of the most pleasurable things was the series of homemade cards Melanie received from one family — a new one came almost every day, with a new handwritten message just for that day. The cards cheered Melanie immensely.

Perhaps the most comforting cards were the ones that wished health and blessings but also suggested that life was going on as usual, something about which Melanie needed to be assured. One day she received a card from a former parishioner from a Chicago church where she had been an interim pastor for nine months. Melanie had liked the woman very much, and the woman had liked Melanie. But after Melanie had left the church, the two hadn't really maintained contact. But Irma had heard of Melanie's illness, and so, seven years after she had last seen her, Irma sent a lovely card that included pictures of her cat and a letter. The letter wasn't earth-shattering in its news; Irma just explained what she had been doing recently. It was the type of letter one might get from a friend one hears from regularly. The tone and the openness of the letter were refreshing; the normality it exuded helped bolster Melanie's spirits. It reminded her that regular life continued outside the hospital room, and that she had friends far removed in place and in time who wanted to let her in on that life. That letter and card were among Melanie's favorites.

The cards had a unique power. Melanie told me that one night when she woke up, there seemed to be a glow in the room. Light poured from the walls papered with the cards. It was, she explained, almost like a mystical experience. Of course, she might not have been awake; it could have been a dream — probably was a dream. Even so, vision or dream (and who can or should distinguish the two?), Melanie experienced a palpable expression of the love the cards carried; in fact, they seemed to carry Melanie herself. It's difficult to express just how much those cards meant to her.

The concept of the communion of saints is simple: people joined over place and time by the love of Christ. And these cards were a marvelous embodiment of that concept: Melanie received cards from people in Indiana, Illinois, Minnesota, Kentucky, North Carolina, Georgia, California, Massachusetts, and possibly other places — I can't quite remember them all. What is extraordinary is that, whether or not the person sending the card knew Melanie, each one said the same thing: we are praying for you. Some offered individual prayers; others indicated that Melanie's name was mentioned during prayer-concern time or printed in the church bulletin so that the entire local congregation could pray for her. And in so doing, in at least one way, these people expressed before the world and to one another their conviction that God listens and that we all matter.

Melanie was glad when she was discharged from the hospital that first time; she had been there a little under one month for her induction therapy, the first cycle in a ten-cycle, almost year-long process. But it saddened her to take her cards down. It was like digging up a beloved garden: perhaps the flowers could be transplanted, but it wouldn't be quite the same. Once she was home, she mentioned several times how much she missed her wall of cards. I kept meaning to try to put them up on a wall of the house, but, as they say, one thing drives out another, and I never got around to it. But I don't think it would have mattered; the mystical wall of cards belonged in the hospital — it wouldn't have been the same duplicated somewhere else. And so there was no wall of cards at home, just a much-revered box of cards.

And the cards continued to come. The news of Melanie's illness took some time to spread, and so, even after the first several months had passed, Melanie continued to receive cards at home from well-wishers who wanted to reach out and express Christian concern. An old seminary professor, a man who had experienced tragedies of his own, wrote a short note expressing his willingness to talk, should Melanie ever want to; he also left it up to Melanie to pursue. She didn't do it; she didn't really have the energy to pursue correspondence. But the offer — knowing that a fellow traveler along life's way who had known great sorrow was available — lifted her spirits. Another note, which arrived some five or six months after her initial hospital stay, came from an old seminary chum whom we hadn't heard from in about eight years. In addition to offering well-wishes, this woman explained the impact Melanie had had on her and Melanie's importance in her life. This note cheered Melanie a great deal.

These notes, cards, and letters circled Melanie's spirit; they represented the white-robed, palm-waving saints of God who shared in her hurt and her healing, her fears and her hopes, her faith and her ambivalence.

Not only was Melanie's spirit buoyed by cards and well-wishes, but our family's physical needs were tended to by local saints. People from our own congregation as well as folks from other churches would bring us meals. This was a particular godsend at first, because Melanie was in the hospital, and I was trying to hold things together — chauffeuring family back and forth, keeping the house intact, and providing comfort for my children. The relief of not having to fix the evening meal was almost like physical nourishment for me; I felt refreshed sitting down to a prepared dinner.

Of course, as nice a thing as this was, it also had its drawbacks. Not because the food wasn't good; it was well made and lovingly delivered. But at times the food hit me like a frying pan in the face because of the other messages it delivered: it wasn't my food; I hadn't fixed it; I hadn't picked out the menu; I had no control. During one stretch of time I thought I would become ill if I had to look at one more meal of spaghetti. The children, as far as I could tell, loved eating spaghetti practically every night. But they were so messy, particularly Gwynne. She couldn't seem to eat spaghetti without getting it all over herself, the table, her chair, and the floor. It was sickening to watch her use her hands to cram fistfuls of spaghetti in her mouth — sometimes to the point where, with her mouth too full to swallow, she had to spit some of the food out. Night after night, it was the same. Red hands and red-stained cheeks and chin. Dried spaghetti strands stuck to the legs of the dining room chairs. Small pieces of meat ground into the floor around her chair. I always tried to clean it up, but she was so messy. And the pots of pasta continued to pour in. At one point, I felt I was sinking in a sea of spaghetti, but I was unable to stem the tide. It kept flowing in because, frankly, I needed it; I had to have something for the kids to eat. At one point, the saints' gift seemed to epitomize my situation: I had no control whatsoever over anything. If one could despair in the midst of kindness, it seemed to me that this was the situation in which that could happen. I appreciated the kindness; I felt part of a very large family. People loved us and showed it. Yet sometimes it all pointed to just how out of joint my life was.

In moments of clarity — removed from the insane situation that cancer produces and the helplessness that it seems to epitomize — I realized just how wonderful the ministrations of the saints were. At times I was overwhelmed by the good that people showed us.

For one thing, a variety of people came to help out or to visit. An old friend from seminary called to say that she was ready to fly out, even though she lived 600 miles away in Virginia. Other friends from graduate school made the 600-mile trip down from Minnesota to spend a weekend with us. Twice we had help from the Chicago area, from families that Melanie had once served as a pastor. Friends came up from Louisville. We were blessed with friends from all around willing to lend a hand. Most of the time I was too reticent to call out for help. But when help was offered, I took it. Folks came in and cooked and cleaned, did the wash and watched the kids. Those visits were very restorative for me: they alleviated what were at times rather dreary periods of unremitting work. Christian charity has taken on a bad image in some circles; I will always hold it out as one of the things that makes it worthwhile to try to hang on to Christianity, warts and all.

Melanie and I had no child care available to us until the fall — so from July (when Melanie was diagnosed) until the first of September, I had to rely on various church members to help with Mave and Gwynne while I stayed with Melanie or tried to put in some time at my job. I tried to rotate requests so that the kids weren't with the same folks more than one time a week, although things didn't always work out that way. Oftentimes Mave and Gwynne were able to spend the day with their little friends; playtime at least helped mask sadtime. A couple of the older women in the church also stayed with the girls. All in all, they were well cared for; those whom they were able to call brother and sister, aunt and uncle, grandma and grandpa were those dear souls in Christ who made themselves available to us as the family of Jesus.

Perhaps the most caring thing the community of saints did for Melanie was to make her feel comfortable about her physical appearance. She did lose her hair because of the chemotherapy. She bought a wig (which she hated), and her mother and sister bought some beautiful scarves and turbans for her to wear. And she did wear them: she wore the wig to church, and the rest of the time when she was out of the house she wore her scarves and turbans. But inside our home she didn't wear a head covering. And all the people who came over or stayed with us supported her in her decision. How? I can't explain it, exactly, except to say that Melanie never felt that she had to run to put on a head covering for these folks.

Melanie heard a story in her cancer-support group that highlighted the importance of this particular blessing. A young woman with cancer had lost her hair, and she told the group that none of her family — not even her husband — had seen her without a wig. She sensed that they would be uncomfortable; she didn't feel that she *could* take the wig off. Maybe it was because such a visible sign would indicate how sick she was; maybe it was because the family really was preoccupied with personal appearance. Whatever the reason, Melanie and I both felt very sorry for this woman. It was sad — she needed support, but she had to mask, in a very real sense, her need.

Our little community of saints accepted Melanie's need, accepted her hair loss, accepted her as she was. There is no greater testimony to the communion of the saints than this — that we are not only a family, but a family of support and love. Christian evangelism would be much easier if all Christian churches embodied what it means to be the community of saints. If they did, then maybe those outside our fellowship would more easily accept our collective baldness and embrace us anyway, to be part of a family of love.

CHAPTER VIII

Walking in Darkness

Even though I walk through the Valley
of Deep Darkness,
I fear no evil; for Thou art with me.

— variant of Psalm 23:4

On July 3, 1991, Melanie and I left for the hospital around 6:30 a.m. We had been told to be there by 7:00 a.m. We had gone shopping the night before to get Melanie things like underwear and pajamas, then packed her overnight bag. We had just about everything we thought she would need; I would later pick up a clock radio with a cassette player. We were there on time; we didn't make it to her room until about 10:00 a.m. This was the first of many reminders that, when it came to Melanie's treatment, things always ran on some other schedule than our own.

Our first experience with the hospital would epitomize much of the journey down medical lane that we would take. A retired man, one of the volunteers, came to take us to

Melanie's room up on the sixth floor, which was, as we would learn, the cancer floor. There was an entire section just for leukemia patients. He escorted us to a room, checked the room number, and then left. And there we were — standing in a room with a big red sign that announced "Bone Marrow Transplant" in black letters. We stood there, we two, staring at each other, afraid to say what was on our minds. Then we began to unpack, nervously filling the drawers and the closet as it all sank in — bone marrow transplant. We weren't ready for it.

And we didn't have to be. Finally, someone explained to us that the rooms reserved for Melanie's type of treatment, an intense cycle of chemotherapy and blood transfusions, had all been full. The rooms were full — no room at the inn. But a room that had been vacated (how, we wondered) would quickly be cleaned, and after a few hours we would find ourselves in a different room, one less sinister because it didn't have that big red sign. Yet, to some degree the damage was done; our suspicions were confirmed. We were not in control, would not be in control, for a long time. We would not pick the rooms or choose the helpers. We would do as we were told, or Melanie would die. And that is what we did throughout the medical process — what we were told. We may have questioned and perhaps even understood things a bit better than the average patient, but the feelings of total dependence and helplessness that descended upon us would not go away.

A modern hospital room and its attendants are very hard to describe. The room is simultaneously cold and warm, friendly and distant, reassuring and terrifying; it involves both routine and surprise. The people most at hand to help — and help they did — were the very ones poking at Melanie throughout the night, making it impossible for her to get a good night's rest. The very personable nurse who stood at her bedside and was so engaging would off-handedly make a very impersonal remark about someone just down the hall, or comment in passing that someone on the floor had died. On one occasion a nurse went so far as to explain to Melanie why she seemed tired and maybe a little grumpy — two people (no names) had died the night before. In trying to give medicine a human face, these individuals also showed a face hardened to dying, and this was the face that always surprised me. I knew that professional distance was important; how else could one survive in a hospital setting? But that understanding didn't take the edges off the harsh reality of seeing people who had gotten used to having others die around them.

That first day, Melanie's oncologist came in to her temporary room to explain to us everything that would be involved, both what the immediate hospital treatment would be like and what would take place later on. All doctors should be like Melanie's — he spent a lot of time with us, and he never seemed to be in a hurry. He made himself present to us. That has been a rare experience for me as a patient and, I think, for Melanie also. But he sat there with us, talking about the nature of the illness, how we would aggressively treat an aggressive disease, and what to expect. And then it all started.

In order to make someone who has acute lymphoblastic leukemia well, you basically have to kill them — at least, kill all their blood cells, hoping, in the process, to kill off all the leukemic cells. Accordingly, Melanie would be fitted with a catheter, and large doses of chemicals would be pumped through it to do the killing. When her blood counts sank down far enough, she would have her red blood cells and her platelets (which assist in blood clotting) replaced through blood transfusions. Then the process of cell murder would begin again. The danger would come with the drop in the white blood cells, which provide the body with protection; they couldn't really be transfused. Oh, in an emergency they could be, but the life cycle of infused white blood cells is only about four hours. So, whereas Melanie's red blood cell count — hemoglobin — and platelet count would drop only to be raised again through transfusion so that she could withstand another onslaught from the chemical killers, it would be different with her white blood cell count — that would continue to drop until, basically, it could drop no further. For all practical purposes, she would be without white blood cells and thus without protection from infection. And if you're worried about infections, the worst place in the world to be is in a hospital, because that's why many of the patients are there.

Melanie's initial stage of treatment — called induction therapy — went extremely well. She was a model patient: she responded well to treatment and aggressively pursued her own care insofar as she could. There was only one period when she became very ill. That happened when the nurse was several hours late in taking her vital signs — this in a situation where signs were typically taken every two hours. Within those few hours, Melanie's temperature shot up. When the nurse eventually discovered the problem, cool cloths were applied to bring down Melanie's fever while tests were sent off to the lab. The results showed that she had picked up both a staph infection and a strep infection. Fortunately, within a day or two, thanks to the wonders of antibiotics, everything was back under control. But, of course, the control was not ours.

After Melanie had been in the hospital just a few days, her environment began to take on an eerie feeling. She was put in protective isolation, which meant that all visitors (mostly limited to family members) had to wash their hands, put on rubber gloves, wear masks, and don sterile gowns. While I was adding to my appearance, at least in a superficial manner, Melanie was shedding aspects of hers — primarily her hair. I was involved in a covering up, she in an uncovering.

Seemingly small things lent at least a modicum of normality to the surroundings. For example, a favorite and greatly anticipated event, as insignificant as it may sound, was our

Sunday-evening viewing of Masterpiece Theater. There we sat at 9:00 p.m. each Sunday night — me dressed up in my isolation outfit, Melanie often fingering her hair to see how much, if any, was coming out — watching together the sordid story of the rise and fall of the household of Augustus Caesar. In some ways, it seemed to mirror our situation — a strong and healthy start to life ends in disintegration. Of course, in *I, Claudius* the decay is moral; in our saga, the decay was physical. Still, the life and death splashed across the screen made me reflect on our living and dying.

The other thing that lent a sense of sanity to Melanie's stay was the letters and stories she wrote for Mave and Gwynne. Mave especially loved to hear stories about herself, particularly stories about when she was born. Before Melanie had gotten sick, she had often taken down the photo albums at home and rehearsed the narrative of life's beginning with Mave. Now, from her hospital bed, Melanie wrote down the story, not only describing the actual events of Mave's birth and the feelings it aroused in us as parents but also, I believe, putting to paper the push for life she herself felt. In affirming Mave's story of creation, she affirmed her own.

> Dear Mave,
>
> We always delighted in telling you about how you were born. Daddy and I were so excited to learn that you were coming. Daddy would sing "Good Morning to You" to my stomach almost every morning. I wanted to name you Miriam, and Daddy wanted to name you Anna Vanessa, so we started calling you MAVEL for Miriam Anna Vanessa Lane. Later on, as we were looking through baby-name books, we saw that Mave was an old Irish name that meant "joy." You were and have been a joy.
>
> I preached as usual on Sunday, rested a lot on Monday — except I had to go back to church to clear up a few things.

On Monday evening, I was having a few contractions off and on — Daddy would only let me have salad for supper. By about 10:00 p.m., I started having these little contractions, 30 seconds long and four to five minutes apart; then contractions a little longer, about two minutes apart. Daddy said I couldn't be in labor because that's not how the book described it, and so he went to bed. About two hours later, I got up and called the doctor, who said, "Ho hum, you might go into the hospital to get checked." So, about one o'clock Tuesday morning, we went in.

The hospital labor room was crowded; we were the last ones in that night, so we were stuck in an exam room and practically forgotten. You didn't take long. Daddy saw your head before the doctor did (she almost missed us). After you were born we got to hold you for a long time, and Daddy sang "Good Morning to You." Also, as you were born, the cassette we had brought to listen to, Gregorian chants, was on its last song, which ended with monastery bells pealing away — perfect timing!

That day you were born was the most special one in my whole life. I love you, Mave.

It was by using little coping devices like these that Melanie made it through her initial hospital stay. More stays would follow, but many fewer than many patients with acute leukemia experience. We made a pact with the oncologist that we would vigorously pursue treatment, insofar as possible, in the confines of his office and in the haven of our home.

The treatment experience took on a different feeling once we were outside the hospital walls. We became responsible for a number of things. For one, Melanie had to spend time each day changing the dressing on her catheter, something that became a ritual of control — this was something she was responsible for and something she could do, and she would do it to the best of her ability. Each day she would remove the old dressing, swab the area with betadine to disinfect it, and prepare a new dressing. Then she would put together the needle she used for flushing her catheter with heparin, a solution that kept the catheter line free of clotted blood. A needle that had to be put together — that surprised me. It was like so many things I learned about during this process. I had no idea — because I had no need to know before — that you could get needles that needed assembly. I had always associated "assembly required" with toys for children that weren't easy to put together. But these were no toys, and they assembled pretty well. Then, once a week, the cliplock for the catheter, the piece attached to the lines through which one pushed the needles, needed to be replaced; this was a two-person job that Melanie and I did together. This ritual made Melanie's illness seem routine.

We administered certain medications at home. The folks from home health care would bring our supplies to us, go over what had to be done, and then leave. Sometimes we just had to use a drip IV to get antiemetics (drugs that controlled nausea) into Melanie before her treatments in the oncologist's office. Once, I remember, the delivery was late, and Melanie had to get her chemo treatment without the antiemetics. It is very frustrating to see someone you love vomiting into a bucket while sitting on the toilet with severe diarrhea because a shipment of medicine is a couple of hours late. But it happened, and we lived with it.

Sometimes Melanie and I did the actual chemotherapy at home, a process that often took a couple of hours to complete. At first we tried to use an IV pump to regulate the flow of medicine. I don't know if we got defective pumps or if they're all ultrasensitive, but we simply couldn't get them to work correctly. We would meticulously set up the line and make absolutely sure there were no air bubbles in it; but then somehow bubbles would appear, and we would end up wrenching the pump open to correct the problem. The pump was extremely sensitive; an air bubble caused it to shut off and give off a warning beep. Finally, the oncologist said the pump really wasn't necessary; we could regulate a gravity-drip IV closely enough without a pump.

Often we would follow up the chemotherapy with a treatment to increase white-cell production in the bone marrow. This procedure called for a hand-held pump that regulated the flow of medicine very precisely. Again, this was always a two-person operation that Melanie and I stumbled through together. We had to put batteries in the pump, prime it, and prepare the line. This process of chemotherapy and white-cell stimulation was repeated every day over about a two-week period. The cost of the drugs: $10,000. There was one month when our pharmacy bill amounted to about $30,000. When one of the local pharmacists who had been filling our less expensive prescriptions commented on how much I was spending on drugs (on one particular day I think it was about $400), I put the cost in context for her. She seemed to be amazed; I still am.

Having Melanie at home was good; doing the drug treatments at home was hard at first. But with practice we became quite proficient at all that had to be done. I generally served as the needle assembler when we did the chemotherapy at home. This treatment usually involved five different needles: three for separate syringes to inject anti-clotting drugs and saline solutions, and two for the IV-catheter connection through which the chemo drugs were administered. Needles used for insertion into catheters are fairly thick as far as needles go. In putting the things together, at first I stuck my fingers with some regularity, which caused two problems: the first was that it hurt like mad because the needles were so thick; the second was that, once I had stuck myself, the needle I was assembling was "contaminated" and no longer usable, and I'd have to start over. But I started over enough times that I finally got the hang of it. In fact, I became so good at it that I was dubbed "Nurse Tom."

But even though we became familiar with the procedures, we never became familiar with the process. In other words, we learned what to do, learned to do it well, and even acted as if it were normal and that we understood all we needed to know about the process — but that process remained radically "other" to us. It was something that was being done to us. We may have known the path to take, but we walked along by touch, not by sight. We still walked in darkness.

Of course, we weren't the only ones walking a path we had not walked before. Surprisingly enough, there were workers in the hospital itself who seemed to be uncomfortable with Melanie and uncertain about how to treat her when she was there. During one visit, the cancer ward was full, so Melanie had to go to an overflow area, a floor that housed mainly heart-surgery patients. When it came time for Melanie's catheter to be flushed, one of the nurses asked her, "Do you know how I'm supposed to do this?" After getting over her initial shock, Melanie took her through the steps of flushing a catheter.

Another strange incident followed. This time Melanie was in dire need of blood; one of the reasons she was in the hospital was that her counts were so low (though she also had a fever, an elevated heart rate, low blood pressure, and a nasty infection in her mouth). But after the first unit of blood was about empty, no one was there to take care of things. Melanie called a nurse. The nurse came in and wondered aloud, "Now how does this get done?" When it became obvious that the nurse was unsure what to do, Melanie guided her through the process of emptying out the entire unit of blood by piggybacking a bag of saline solution; that way the saline washed down all the blood and cleared the IV lines of blood so that clotting wouldn't be a problem. The last straw came when Melanie was being injected with antibiotics through her catheter: the attendant never swabbed the catheter head with alcohol. Melanie expressed both dismay and concern: What was going on?

As it turned out, Melanie was on the floor that trained a large number of student nurses. Several of those attending Melanie did not in fact know what to do with her. But they were never identified as student nurses: they didn't wear ID tags, nor did they tell Melanie that they were students. Training students in the medical professions is fine; we had no problem with that. But it would have been nice to know, up front, who they were and what to expect (which was a lot of "I don't know" looks and uncertainty about what to do). This made it clear to us yet again that not only did we lack a firm grasp of the treatment process itself, but we often didn't know anything about who was treating Melanie and if they were qualified to do so. Most were; some weren't. It made an already uncertain situation even more uncertain.

Psalm 23, probably the most beloved and most well-known psalm in our time, has a line that reads, "Yea, though I walk through the Valley of the Shadow of Death, I will fear no evil, for thou art with me." This line from the King James Version emphasizes — at least the way it is heard — the notion of death. It is true that God is with us even in the borderland of death. But I recently noticed a textual variant of this verse that better described my feelings at the time. It goes like this: "Yea, though I walk through the Valley of Deep Darkness . . ." This psalm affirms that God is with us, not just at the time of death but in all dark times.

Melanie and I were walking through a deep darkness. It was as if someone had dropped us in the middle of an ancient, hoary forest, with trees so high and full that they blocked out the sun. A forest so dense that even at noontime the forest floor was dusky, shadowy at best. A forest that was cool, damp, and powerful in its dimness. Sometimes I feel that we were dropped down in the middle of that forest at twilight, so that it was already becoming quite dark within its confines. Not totally dark — we could still make out the forms of trees, the various fungi growing through the moist ground, maybe see rock foundations and a stream of dark, lively water. But it was getting dark. Soon we wouldn't be able to make out even these things. We would know they were there, but the pitch blackness of the forest night would create an impenetrable blanket of unseeing. And I knew that it was through that unseeing that we would have to walk. We would get our bearings before dark, make out the forms in the shadowland. But soon, soon, I knew that, mentally and spiritually, we would be walking forward, perhaps following the sound of hope the flowing stream made, but in darkness. We would know vaguely what was in front of us, but in the darkness we would stumble forward. We would walk through the deep darkness of life, hoping to come out into the daylight of better life.

At one time or another, we all walk through this forest. The stream is God's Word to us, that which leads us through the deep darkness, that which gives hope to our hopelessness and help to our helplessness. The Word made flesh, Jesus Christ, is the presence of God with us in the forest of deep darkness. And, all together, we hope to make it through.

In our situation, hope was the operative word. We hoped to make it through. The tangle of IV pole trees, with their leafy bags of chemicals, cut us off from the sunlight, yet we had hope. Hope not only to understand but to survive the deep darkness. Hope that the deep darkness was not bane but protection from an even deeper and worse darkness. And we walked not by sight but by faith: by faith — as much as we could muster — in the treatments and in the doctors and nurses and other medical personnel; by faith — as much as we could call upon — in ourselves to keep walking, to continue to fight, to stretch our hands out in front of us as we stumbled along; by faith in a God who not only walked along with us in our darkness but who shared our darkness. One who himself hung on a cross under a dark sky, a deep darkness of sin and evil and hurt and finitude.

We walked along, Melanie and I. And the point is that we continued. We did walk. Flannery O'Connor once said that faith is a walking in darkness, not a theological solution to mystery. Both Calvin and Luther affirmed a hidden God. Though they may have meant something different by the phrase, I like it. The hidden God. One who is not apparent to our senses; one who hides from our inquiries and attempts to find him. But a hidden God who is up just ahead, in the deep darkness, moving from tree to tree, with a voice that beckons us onward, calling on us to affirm life and its goodness despite the darkness. God is not something one comes up with as a solution; he is the one up ahead, calling faintly, like a whip-poorwill at dusk. God is the hidden one who gives us courage to follow after the voice, trusting it to lead us one day out of deep darkness into the daylight of his heavenly kingdom. We trust, we walk in darkness, and hope that indeed what is ahead is open field and not bottomless abyss.

CHAPTER IX

Rightful Minds

Dear Lord and Father of mankind,
Forgive our foolish ways!
Reclothe us in our rightful mind,
In purer lives Thy service find,
In deeper reverence, praise.

—John Greenleaf Whittier, 1872

One of the problems with dealing with any sort of cancer, it seems to me, is that the physical aspects of coping are so entirely encompassing that you don't get around to dealing with the mental aspects of the disease until you're already in some degree of difficulty. This is not simply a matter of "accepting" your illness, although that has to be done. But once you accept it, you can get so caught up, if you're the sick person, in treatment plans, medical routines, visits to the doctor, and so on that you're too busy to pay much attention to how you feel about what's going on and how it's affecting you as you. If you're the helper of a cancer-stricken person, you're caught up to some degree in the same sorts of things: driving to the doctor, helping out with the medical procedures, dealing with the physical reactions to the treatment. On top of that, the helper has to take on other, added duties: extra child care, the entire load of household chores, and, perhaps worst of all, the nightmare of insurance reimbursement. Then there's the monthly task of balancing the checkbook, trying to figure out who you can rob to pay off someone else. When prescription drugs run hundreds and hundreds of dollars each month, a check that comes in two months later as a reimbursement isn't always a lot of help. Immersed in this sea of tasks, the helper has no time to think, "Hey, how do I feel about all this? Am I coping? What is this doing to me?" And so, in your busyness, in a real sense you forget about yourselves to an extent, forget about the "me" inside the sick person's body and the "me" inside the helper's body.

Just naming the disease is often the hardest thing to do. In our minds, we sometimes think that if we don't name something, it isn't real. We avoid the issue. "Cancer" was the big word for Melanie and for all of us in her family. In some way, at least at first, we all avoided the term. We did say "leukemia"; most often I said "acute lymphoblastic leukemia." What usually happened after I articulated the entire name of Melanie's disease was that, since I had chosen to say a mouthful, I would have to take the time to define the words to whomever I was talking. That gave me a chance to be the diagnostician, to explain to everyone else what the whole thing meant. And, after the first few days, I got pretty good at this: I could spend a lot of time unpacking the terms. It was a safe thing to do. It put distance between me and the disease, to speak so objectively about what it was that was ravaging my wife's body.

Melanie's mom was much the same way. She avoided talking directly about what it was Melanie had. I think that she, as I did, felt safer behind the bigger words — they had impact, but less of an emotional impact than the much smaller, simpler, and for some reason more menacing word "cancer." Melanie was the first one to actually start using the word. As with so many things, Melanie was the most frank, most take-charge person when it came to her health and understanding not only the physical but also the emotional issues involved.

Nevertheless, even Melanie was a bit evasive at first when she talked about her cancer — that ugly word that carries more negative connotations in our collective minds, I think, than any other illness. Her avoidance showed up in her early conversations on the phone and in the first letter she wrote to her congregation. In neither case, that first week or two, did she say "I have cancer." She always phrased it in the third person: "The preacher has cancer." It was curious to me that she would put it that way. Frequently the context was one in which she was trying to assure a church member that everything would be OK or telling the church that things would go on as usual. She would say things like, "I don't want the church to stop doing things just because the preacher has cancer." The preacher has cancer. But eventually it dawned on her that she was the preacher and that she had the cancer. So her use of the noun gave way to her use of the first-person pronoun: "I have cancer." That was a hard and scary thing to say.

Melanie's mother, who visited often, even expressed a little hostility when Melanie started saying "cancer." It was late afternoon, I remember, and her mother and I were making our way home from the hospital on the back roads of rural Indiana, driving by the rows and rows of corn that would eventually burn up that summer because of the heat and lack of rain. "Well," her mother said, "I guess you heard that she's using the 'c' word." The "c" word; Melanie was using it, and she had it. And Melanie's mom didn't like to hear it. Why should she? It is a word that can strike at our deepest fears, prick the skin of our finitude, and show us our lifeblood running out. All that in a single word. I didn't like the word, either. Melanie was braver than both her mom and me when it came to looking fear in the eye and facing it down. Getting acquainted with the word "cancer" was symbolic of our getting our minds acquainted with the problem at hand. It was an ill-received visitor.

If the word "cancer" was not welcome, neither were some of the doctors we had to deal with; they made Melanie's mental anguish worse, not better. Her oncologist, as I've said before, was great. He always took a lot of time to explain things to her, and he remained upbeat about Melanie's medical profile and her chances of making it through the treatment and getting well. This helped Melanie have a positive attitude toward much of her chemotherapy. But her radiologist took a very different approach.

Melanie's really severe mental anxiety began with her radiation therapy. On the surface of it, there shouldn't have been anything to be afraid of. She was to be given "brain treatments": her entire brain area would receive relatively low doses of X-ray therapy for a relatively short period of time — less than a minute per brain side. She would need only ten treatments — less than twenty minutes' total radiation therapy over a two-week period. This therapy was important because the drugs that fight leukemia have a hard time penetrating brain tissue because of its peculiar makeup. Leukemic cells can, in a real sense, "hide out" in the brain while most are killed off in the rest of the body. Relapses come primarily from those hidden bad cells. Recovery rates for leukemic patients have increased greatly since the discovery of this fact. All in all, radiation therapy should have been seen as a good thing working for Melanie's total recovery.

Unfortunately, Melanie's radiologist wasn't at all like her oncologist. He made a point of telling her that there was at least the possibility of mental incapacitation due to the treatment. The possibility was slight, he said, but there was a chance she could suffer some side effect — short-term or long-term. That warning would have been enough. But he went on and on about it. He talked about how, in children, there most definitely is a problem: the X rays adversely affect their brain cells because they haven't fully matured. Of course, since Melanie was an adult, the treatment probably wouldn't hurt her — but it could. It could. He must have said "it could" ten times or more. And by the time he was finished with her, Melanie was very afraid. Afraid of losing her mind. Afraid of losing mental capacity. Afraid of not being able to read or think or preach sermons.

As a consequence, Melanie came to dread her radiation therapy more than anything else in her treatment. Perhaps unconsciously or unthinkingly, this doctor destroyed in ten minutes the self-confidence that Melanie's oncologist had tried to build up over a period of five weeks. For the first time, Melanie began to cry when it came time for her radiation treatment. And so, the radiologist joined several other people I had to deal with over the next year or so of Melanie's fight for life. They were decidedly unhelpful in the way they affected the mental preparedness and toughness required of both Melanie and me to wage the battle we had on our hands.

The healing process may or may not in part depend on a patient's mental attitude. Some studies indicate that it does; others vigorously deny that psychology plays a part in physical healing. Part of what it means to be religious, I think, is to believe that such factors as faith do play an important part in the healing process. Not in terms of a simple "Just believe and everything will be fine"; that is a blatant lie, one that needs to be wiped off the smirky faces of self-righteous ministers and Christians who are ill-prepared to respond meaningfully to sickness. The people I had the most trouble with during Melanie's treatment were the unthinking Christians who blandly smile through life's problems (if they have had any) and throw out to those in trouble an insidious "Give thanks in all things" or "God works for the good of them who love him." In my case, that was like throwing a cement block to a drowning person. There was the un-Christian assumption in so much of this talk that real Christians don't have life-threatening problems if they believe hard enough, or that those circumstances are somehow insignificant for the "person of faith." That kind of assumption suggested that there was something wrong with my faith or my wife's faith — which, of course, there was. On his deathbed, Martin Luther said, "We are all beggars. It is true." Even in our faith, we beg for more, because what we have is inadequate. But everyone's faith is inadequate; we should support one another rather than hold each other to standards none can meet.

And there came a time when Melanie needed a lot of support for her mental well-being, both psychological support and physical support in the form of drugs.

A little less than two months after Melanie was discharged from that initial hospital stay in the summer of 1991, she began to experience a letdown. Her oncologist had warned her that it would come. In the hospital, you have lots of support and, frankly, everything is still new — you're still in the process of trying the disease on for size. The game you're playing is dead serious — life or death — but you're also fascinated, in a way, with learning about the various procedures and drugs, what everything is supposed to do, how you're going to "act" as a sick person. Then you go home, and going home is a great relief. You're with family and friends again. But then, about a month into the process at home, you begin to understand that your sickness is going to stay with you for quite a while. The newness wears off. You get sick of being sick. And, inevitably, depression sets in.

It hit Melanie quite suddenly. It was Labor Day, and her folks had flown up for the weekend. Melanie became distrustful and a bit confused. She kept pulling me aside for "reality checks." The things her mother was saying in the living room — were they true? Were people lying to her? Melanie told me that after practically every sentence she had heard, she had said to herself, "That's a lie."

I was concerned. I would have been even more concerned had I known that she also disbelieved most of what I was saying. My father had recently retired, and so he and my mother had gone on a grand tour of the country, covering about 10,000 miles round trip. So I shared details of my folks' travels with my in-laws — where they had been and how long it had taken them to get there and how no place was as beautiful as the north Georgia mountains where they lived. As it turned out, Melanie sat there the entire time thinking that I was making the whole thing up — that my parents were not on a trip, that my father had not retired — and wondering why I was lying that way.

Of course, we quickly brought the situation to the attention of Melanie's oncologist; Melanie found the disorientation and the hideous sense of mistrust she felt to be almost as bad as or worse than the leukemia.

The oncologist assured Melanie that she wasn't going out of her mind — which is what Melanie had become particularly afraid of, thanks to the radiologist prating on about mental incapacitation as a possible consequence of radiation therapy. Then the doctor asked her several key questions, focusing especially on her sleeping habits. His diagnosis was clinical depression. He emphasized that this did not mean simply that Melanie felt "blue," although that feeling can coincide with clinical depression. Rather, he said, the problem was in the chemistry of the brain: during times of great stress, the chemical processes of the brain get somewhat skewed, so that there can be a lack of serotonin, something the brain needs for proper rest. Lack of REM (rapid eye movement) sleep is an indicator that serotonin is not being produced in sufficient amounts. Given his diagnosis, the doctor started Melanie on an antidepressant drug, gradually increasing the dosage until it gave her maximum benefit. Melanie began to sleep much better, and most of her feelings of distrust and disorientation disappeared.

I told some people about Melanie's depression and its treatment, and I wish I hadn't. In fact, I soon stopped talking about it altogether. It was apparent that many of the people I mentioned this to seemed to somehow or other blame the depression on a lack of will in Melanie — that she was somehow deficient for being depressed, or that it was a "mood" that a "normal" person certainly could control. Talk about neural transmitters seemed to do little good; there was an obvious stigma attached to depression, and it surprised the hell out of me.

I was even more surprised when the depression hit me. It wasn't surprising to Melanie's oncologist, but it was to me — and embarrassing, especially after I had witnessed the prejudicial judgments hurled at Melanie for her depression. My God, I thought, I'm not even sick. What will they think? They thought nothing, of course, because I told only one person outside my family.

Given that I literally earn my keep by speaking — as a teacher and a preacher — it was ironic that the prospect of explaining my condition to Melanie's oncologist was so embarrassing that I was almost rendered speechless. But I got started by telling him about the signs I had noticed: waking up a lot at night, being very tired in the morning, getting light-headed, and being unable to concentrate at work. He asked a few follow-up questions, and then asked a very simple question: When you wake up at night to go to the bathroom, do you have to wait for an erection to go down to go? I was confused and embarrassed by the question. What did that have to do with anything? But, in fact, I never had to wait for an erection to go down to urinate. Then the doctor told me that that was a very simple way of telling if a male was suffering from clinical depression — an obvious sign. Men have erections during REM sleep; no erections, no REM. The doctor immediately prescribed medicine for me and then referred me to an internist who would take care of me during this time of crisis in my life. After a few nights on the medicine, I began to feel much better — rested in a way I had not for several months. In terms of at least the chemically controlled portion of my own mental problems, the medicine was a godsend.

But in probing my mental state, the doctor hit on another area hard for me to discuss (or write about) because I am a naturally reticent person. He wanted to know how Melanie and I were doing sexually. So I explained, from my vantage point, that it was difficult sometimes. Melanie and I tried to carry on some semblance of a sex life, but she was sick, and I was so tired all the time. I think both of us felt diminished desire. Psychologically, we knew it was important to try to maintain the intimacy of making love, but physical and mental weariness often stood in the way.

It's funny how the mind works and what it remembers. When my students read or talk about St. Augustine's *Confessions,* some of them find it interesting that Augustine remembered so vividly a single event from his past — stealing pears from a pear tree — and that he explored how that event shaped his life and theology. They sometimes think it stretches things a bit to put so much emphasis on a simple childhood occurrence, which more than likely shouldn't even warrant remembering. But remember Augustine's mind did. And it was this sort of memory that began to invade my mind and my thoughts about sex during the times Melanie and I were intimate.

When I was thirteen, we lived for a summer with my grandmother. For the first time I was beginning to explore my sexuality fully, which brought with it my initial episodes of masturbation. Since I attended a highly moralistic Baptist church, I both physically enjoyed the pleasure while at the same time I felt that there was something terribly wrong with doing it. Those two things combined to make my times alone in the bathroom times of terrified enjoyment. I imagined God at the Last Judgment, calling me before the mighty host. Then, just like at a drive-in movie, my life would be flashed up on a giant screen; all my private times would be made public before the judgment throne. This may sound silly. It is also an awful depiction of God and his judgment, but one that was all too real to me (and still is for many).

This is the memory that came back to plague me, because one of the ways that Melanie and I tried to maintain sexual activity was by having Melanie lie beside me and talk to me while I masturbated. This gave us a sense of closeness and sexuality that didn't tax Melanie's strength — and, since I was really tired much of the time, it was also easier for me physically than intercourse. But mentally it was very difficult. Besides all the psychological hang-ups that one normally might be aware of while masturbating in the presence of another, I was haunted by that vivid picture which had originated in my early adolescence — God watching me masturbate. There were times when I couldn't reach orgasm, or climaxed only after a very long time, because this image kept lurking in the corners of my mind.

And so, even in the attempts that Melanie and I made to gain intimacy in the way best suited to our situation, God crept in; and it still puzzles me that this picture of God, one that I thought I had long abandoned, appeared at this point with such clarity. Sex and a vengeful God — maybe it meant that, during our most private moments, I still saw God in some sense as an enemy of the goodness of life. The image that at times seemed to crush my sex drive may have haunted my thoughts because a part of me, the deepest part, thought that God was trying to crush Melanie and me altogether. So this peculiar connection between my childhood, our sex life, and God became part of the equipment that I used in my daily mental gymnastics as I tried to balance all my feelings and thoughts about God and God's place in what was going on.

Mave and Gwynne, of course, worked through their own kind of mental anguish. They obviously did it in different ways, being affected differently by what was going on around them. Since Gwynne was only two, we couldn't really explain to her what was happening, and she couldn't use language to say how she felt. And although Melanie and I would occasionally try to talk to Mave about what was going on, even she, at five, was really too young to understand it in a verbal way, or to express in clearly connected sentences what she was feeling and what scared her and how she was coping. These things came out primarily during the girls' playtime.

During one of those playtimes, I overheard something that made me feel both completely shocked and completely unsurprised at the same moment; it sounds impossible, but that was the combination of feelings I had. I was listening to the girls play with their Barbie dolls. Mave, who was in charge of setting up the playtime scenario, coolly and calmly said to Gwynne, "Pretend our mommy died and we're left by ourselves. And pretend I'm the big sister who has to take care of you." And so the Barbies entered the world of orphanhood, exploring what it was like to be without a mommy, having only each other to rely on.

I was shocked because, for the first time, Mave expressed quite forcefully all of her fears as well as ours. I couldn't believe my ears. She was actually playing out Melanie's death in Barbie's world. It was unnerving.

At the same time, I wasn't surprised, because I know that children often act out their feelings during playtime. As a matter of fact, I had expected that at some point the possibility of Melanie's death would come up during their fantasy time. I expected it — but that's not the same thing as hearing it for the first time. Melanie and I never discouraged the girls from exploring this possibility in play; it was, after all, one of their few emotional outlets for what was going on inside them. Still, it was odd to listen to as it became a more and more frequent focus of their playtime, not just with their Barbies but in other play situations as well.

I tried not to dwell too much on the fact that, in their play, Mommy's death meant orphanhood. After all, I would still be around. What orphanhood may have represented to them, however, was the extreme instability of the situation and the way it made them feel — insecure. If Mommy could die, then so could Daddy. Melanie and I even tried at times (mostly near the end of her treatment) to assure them that, even if something did happen to one or both of us, they would be taken care of by people who loved them — they wouldn't be orphans. I wanted to say, "I'll be around. I'll never die." But under the circumstances, not only would that have been a lie of sorts — how could I promise something like that? — but it would not have alleviated the real root of their mental anguish: the intrusion of the real possibility of finitude into their young lives. Just as Melanie and I had to deal with this fact, they did too. And they explored it through the idea of orphanhood.

And when Melanie and I talked with a therapist about Mave and about the kinds of things she liked to watch on the VCR, the two of us realized that she — as well as Gwynne — were exploring orphanhood in other ways, too. For the entire period of Melanie's illness, Mave and Gwynne's favorite videos were *Annie* and the Shirley Temple movies. Annie, of course, is an orphan. And in every Shirley Temple movie we've seen, Shirley always plays an orphan.

Melanie and I found that much of our mental anguish had to do with matters of faith. And the fear of orphanhood — a more fundamental orphanhood — sometimes seized us too. Had we been orphaned by God? Sometimes it seemed like it. Were we God's children, beloved of God? It sometimes seemed like that, too. "Dear Lord and Father of mankind," Whittier had written, ". . . reclothe us in our rightful mind." I think Melanie and I both knew that, in order to regain our minds, we would have to, in some sense, feel more like children than orphans. We were struggling in a balancing act, and we hoped that the sense of orphanhood would not eventually tip the scales.

CHAPTER X

Holiday Hope

I wonder as I wander out under the sky,
Why Jesus the Savior did come for to die
For poor onr'y sinners like you and like I.
I wonder as I wander out under the sky.

— John Jacob Niles, 1960

On this day earth shall ring
with the song children sing
to the Lord Christ our King,
born on earth to save us,
him the father gave us.

— 1582; translated by
Jane Marion Joseph

And his name shall be called Emmanuel,
which means, God with us.

— Matthew 1:23b

Melanie had been very ill around the week of Thanksgiving and had had to go back to the hospital, though by Thanksgiving Day itself she was feeling better. I took her a Thanksgiving meal, one that I had bought ahead of time at the local grocery store. For heat-and-serve Thanksgiving, it was pretty good. Still, we had made big plans for that day, with my parents coming to visit. So it was a disappointment that Melanie couldn't be home to share the good food and family togetherness.

But Christmastime was much different. Despite its commercialization, there's something *real* about Christmas. I once read an article by Andrew Greeley in which he makes a keen observation: that probably at least half of what Christians know about their faith they learn around the crèche scenes set up at Christmastime. I don't think that's a bad thing, because it shows us a God who comes in swaddling clothes. Easter may be, theologically, the most important concept of Christianity. But it is Christmastime that makes it all seem real and believable because you have a real and believable baby to look at and admire. The Incarnation means more than God looking like us for a while, but it is at least that, and that is probably what makes Christianity, as far as it is understandable, intelligible to most folks. God does seem to be with us at Christmastime.

What's more, Christmas balances quite nicely the very real with the miraculous (or, some would say, the mythological; I don't think it much matters, because the truly and enduringly mythological is a miracle all its own). There's the cast of characters, so real that they could just as easily be people we know as characters from a story. There's Mary, the young girl, both astounded and frightened by the upcoming birth, not unlike any young woman facing childbirth for the first time, God involved or not. There's stolid Joseph, who stands by, giving his grudging support, pushed into his responsibilities toward Mary by God's assurances — again, not unlike the many young men who need a nudge to fulfill their responsibilities in the role of father. A clever medieval English Christmas song that I like may give away more about Joseph than the Bible allows, but it doesn't seem like an unfair characterization. Mary asks Joseph to pick a cherry from the cherry tree for her and the baby. (Remember that the medieval English didn't really know that the Middle East grows precious few cherry trees.) Joseph's curt reply is, "If you and your baby want a cherry, why don't you ask the father to get it?" Of course, the baby Jesus in the womb commands the cherry branches to bend down to Mary, but you get the point — Joseph isn't all holiness and goodness and forgiveness, as no real human being is. He's peevish, just as we all are at times.

Then there's the grubby innkeeper, pushing out a young married couple, claiming he has no more room — though there's always room if there's enough money. And, of course, the whole story is in a way centered around that most human of inventions — taxes. Census figures weren't being compiled just so Roman bureaucrats could juggle precinct lines. In short, the Christmas story is a very real story, full of honest-to-goodness human characters, that happens to throw in the birth of the son of God along with everything else. And here's the real miracle: God's Incarnation comes in a very natural way — through childbirth — to a very natural couple in a natural setting, an impoverished one for the poor young folks. And it's how God comes to us still: in our everyday, ordinary lives as we go about doing and being subjected to everyday, ordinary things.

For me, and I think for Melanie too, the Christmas season became a season of hope precisely because of all that undergirds the Christmas tradition: God coming to us in a human way through human ways. And we were expectant that God would come to us in our very human predicament — facing finitude and trying not to let it overwhelm us.

It turned out to be a joyful Christmastime. Melanie had her heart set on having a good holiday season, and so did I. It seems we were invigorated — inspired, really — to have a good Christmas. Melanie, in fact, made a declaration: Christmas would be better and happier than Thanksgiving. Though joy is at times spontaneous, there's something to be said for those who willfully pursue it, dogging it by dint of volitional efforts. And that's what we did. And we were joyful and, for at least part of the time, sure of God's presence that makes happy the sorrowful.

In many ways, the whole of the season was symbolized for me by our shopping for and then putting together a Christmas tree. We decided to get an artificial tree. The church had used one the year before, and it had looked very nice, nothing like the chintzy-looking silver aluminum trees that I remembered from my childhood. In years past, we had always dragged home a live tree. But then we would discover that it had a hole in the greenery we hadn't noticed before. Or that it was crooked at the very bottom, and so we would have to figure out how to cut off the bottom without sawing off too much. Or that the tree's top was somehow wrong and we'd have to try to fix it so the star would stay on. So this year we decided to go for prepackaged beauty. We wanted to buy a tree that would be beautiful in its completeness. And off we went.

We actually ended up looking at several different stores on several different occasions. Apparently, the worldwide artificial-Christmas-tree industry had decided to make only one tree that was as beautiful as the one I had seen. So we had to comparison shop. Store after store, none of the trees we saw looked quite right. Finally, we chose one that everyone except Mave liked the best. Although it wasn't completely beautiful, it was a nice-looking artificial tree.

Besides beauty, however, I sought something dearer, really, to my heart — ease. I had figured that an artificial tree would be a snap to put together. Haul the branches out of the box, stick them in the post, and voila! — instant beauty. This seemed like it would be so much simpler than tromping off to a Christmas tree farm, finding the one tree we thought would be perfect (but wouldn't be) at the very back of the lot, and trudging it through the mud (why is it always muddy at Christmas tree farms?) to the front of the acreage to pay for it. Then there was the whole ordeal of getting the tree home, prepping it, and coaxing it to actually stand up. Yes, an instant tree held out the promise of carefree assembly. I honestly bought an artificial tree because I thought it would be both beautiful and easy. And it was beautiful.

But after the first two hours, it began to dawn on me that putting the tree together wasn't going to be quite as easy as I had imagined. After four hours, I was pretty sure it wasn't. Branches had to be unfolded and unbent, matched, and put together in the right order. I was almost positive that the tree from our box was defective; there was no way I could get it to look like the tree displayed in the store.

But I kept trying, with encouragement (and razzing) from the family. Finally, I got the tree put together, every last set of matched branches. And it was pretty. And it had been much harder than I had thought it would be. In its artificial way, it symbolized what we were really going through. Our Christmas season living with the threat of leukemic annihilation was beautiful and meaningful, but it didn't just happen. We had to work at it. At times, it was hard to put together a tree of Christmas joy in the face of difficult circumstances. But we persevered, kept our goal in mind, and a joyful Christmas took shape through our plodding efforts.

One of the mainstays of my faith during the Christmas season was a song. I had always liked the song; the version done by King's College Choir, Cambridge, made it one of my favorites. But during this particular holiday season it was more than a favorite song — it was a sustaining song, giving what at times seemed palpable support to me in my efforts to join with my family in a bond of divine love from whence we believed true joy would spring:

Of the Father's heart begotten,
e're the world from chaos rose.
He is Alpha; from that fountain
all that is and hath been flows.
He of all things is Omega
yet to come the mystic close,
evermore and evermore.

This song about Jesus builds as it makes its way through various verses until it reaches the final, ringing stanza that has heaven and all its beings, countless in number, singing Christ's praises "evermore and evermore."

There's a majesty and a completeness to the song in the way it describes the inevitable course of God's love for us and the praise due Christ for his gift of love to us. Put this song together with a verse or two of "Away in a Manger," and the magic of Christmas is neatly presented: the majesty and the manger, the miraculous and the mundane, the divine and the human all joined as one giant symbol that, despite its commercialization, still stands as one of the clearest presentations of God with us. As John Calvin put it, the Incarnation shows us a God who is near us, not far away.

One of the best things about Christmas, with its emphasis on "God with us," is that the divine closeness of the heavenly family is mirrored in the gathering of earthly families at this time. In our mobile society, with families scattered like so much buckshot across the country, Christmas still serves to bring families back together. Despite its schmaltziness, the song "I'll Be Home for Christmas" does say something important: even when we're not physically with our families during Christmas, emotionally we are — or at least we long to be. Christmas captures a yearning many of us have for at least one day a year when memories of being with family and friends can be cherished, or when new memories can be made.

Melanie's folks came up from Georgia for Christmas. This was a source of tremendous excitement for our kids and for us. The emphasis was on being together, so we didn't spend a lot of time in the kitchen; on Christmas Day we had a heat-and-serve feast (though a passable one, complete with a honey-smoked ham). That time had a eucharistic feeling for me, in the sense of portending unity over space and time, as the Eucharist does. In our church, one of the standard liturgies announces, "Friends, this is the joyful feast of the people of God. They will come from east and west, and north and south, to sit at table together in the kingdom of God." In its simplicity, this liturgy paints a compelling and achingly beautiful portrait of life together with God. And it suggests much the same feeling I had with family who came from hundreds of miles away to visit. Prior to my in-laws' advent from Georgia, my sister had come through town on her way to visit my other sister — from El Paso, Texas, to Washington, D.C., through Indianapolis, Indiana. We pretty much had east and west and north and south wrapped up that December.

Church was wonderful during the Advent season. One Advent Sunday, Melanie preached one of the best sermons I had ever heard her give. Afterward, the person sitting in front of me commented that Melanie could say more in fifteen minutes than most people could in an hour, and for this sermon, at least, that was true. Our little choir offered much special music that was both beautiful and inspiring in its content and its presentation. And the Sunday before Christmas there was a fellowship time after church, during which the church presented Melanie with a card stuffed with money (more than we would have imagined) and a handmade wreath, both signs of the church's concern and care for Melanie. Melanie cried, and I was touched; even now the wreath hangs prominently in the dining room.

Few things can compare with a Christmas Eve service, particularly if it's a simple one. We read the Christmas story in short snippets, sang carols as a congregation, and enjoyed lots of special music — I sang "Silent Night" in the original (*Stille Nacht*) accompanied only with a guitar. And, of course, we ended with a candle-lighting ceremony. The chilling, austere beauty of the Indiana night was matched by the simple beauty of the service. I can think of few services of worship as meaningful as that one: in the cold of winter, life was affirmed; and in the cold reaches of my soul, a spark was fanned into a fire that kept the darkness at bay.

Finally, there was Santa Claus. On Christmas Eve he actually came to our house, all dressed in fur. Mave and Gwynne were delighted; they even got warm-up presents to prepare them for Christmas Day. Santa was his jolly self, and he made sure he listened to every wish, though promising nothing (a smart Santa!). There are people who think Santa is a very bad influence on kids; I remember when one well-known TV curmudgeon, in commenting on the Santa phenomenon, said that kids should be told the truth. Specifically, he wanted to correct the guy who wrote little Virginia long ago declaring, "Yes, Virginia, there is a Santa Claus." There's enough delusion already, he said. Tell Virginia the truth. What he said next shocked me: "There's too much childlike trust in the world." If he meant this statement literally, or if it's taken that way, I think it comes as close to the demonic as I'm willing to admit exists in our world.

For here's the whole point and, for me, the whole connection between Christmas and Santa: childlike trust. If Christmas, in all its crass materialism and self-indulgent fits of buying frenzy, can still somehow or other evoke within us a sense of wonder and childlike trust, I am more than willing to tolerate it; I will celebrate it. Christmas, at its best and despite its worst, opens our eyes to a new world, a new world on the verge of this world — indeed, a new world ushered in through all the inanities of the old. But to see the vision, it takes the sight of a trusting child. It is the vision the prophets call for; it is the hope we all yearn for.

My favorite Christmas story is Dr. Seuss's *How the Grinch Stole Christmas.* There's that marvelous part of the narrative when, hearing the Whos singing on Christmas morning despite their lack of presents, the Grinch has a change of heart; actually, he has a changed heart — it goes from being too small to being three times as large as normal. The TV adaptation of the book adds that, as a result of this growth, the Grinch had the strength of "ten grinches, plus two."

I wondered about a lot of things because of Melanie's sickness. In my wanderings, I wondered about God and about what the Christmas story said to me. But beneath my wondering, deeper than my knowing, was my feeling, and my feeling was enlarged by the Christmas story. The manger made me a stronger, better person, more trusting in God and in the goodness of life, despite life's attempts to wreck the good and the Godly. I heard the song of Christmas, and my heart grew; I felt true joy; I felt I had the strength of ten plus two.

Despite Melanie's illness, during this Christmas I was made bold to join in song: "On this day earth shall ring/ with the song children sing." I was a bell that rang, resonating Christmas glory, sounding its gladness. And, in my hope, I hoped Melanie heard me, and joined me.

CHAPTER XI

To Sing Again

(The Mystery of Living)

God made life a gamble,
and we're still in the game.

— country singer Joe Diffie

In heavenly love abiding,
no change my heart shall fear.
And safe is such confiding,
for nothing changes here.
The storm may roar without me,
my heart may low be laid.
But God is round about me,
and can I be dismayed?

— hymn by Anna Waring, 1850

It would be nice if life could be neatly categorized — better yet, if the neat categories actually worked in lived experience. But, when all is said and done, there remains an intractable ambiguity in life that resists attempts to make it into either a crapshoot or an airtight certainty — that is, in religious terms, which are the only terms that, for me, come close to at least laying bare the meaning of all that ambiguity.

I ponder that ambiguity more nowadays, though not in a morbid (not most days, anyway) manner. I'm more reflective now, partly because I have the time to be reflective. As I write these pages today, Melanie requires much less care. What I have compressed into these few chapters occurred over a period of about a year. From the time of our Christmas celebration to the end of Melanie's treatment plan was about four months. Nothing stands out during those months that I haven't handled thematically already. It was simply four more months of the same: hope and despair, God's presence and God's absence, dog-tiredness and little moments of everyday grace. Those elements remain now, but in a less pressing way, with a different flavor. Being on the "finished" end of the treatment doesn't make all my questions go away, but I can think about them in a more leisurely manner — though not any less seriously.

Melanie was a model patient throughout her treatment; she was a favorite of many nurses and, I suspect, of her oncologist. She turned out to be a stunning example of how well everything could work. She is in full remission after aggressively pursuing her health in what was, actually, an extremely close to textbook round of treatment — she actually beat the "idealized" goal for treatment length by about a month. (Most folks, because of physical or emotional problems, have to have the schedule adjusted, slowed down, as it were.) I am very proud of Melanie, and very glad that she seems to have won her battle with leukemia.

Of course, a number of questions still remain. Why did it have to happen? What have we learned from it? Should we have *had* to learn anything from so terrible an experience? The religious question that is foremost for me in many ways has to do with God's role in this entire process — and that, of course, remains a carefully balanced ambiguity.

Does God just create things and let them fly, let them run of their own accord? Did God in fact make life a gamble? There were times when this seemed very much to be the case. There was no apparent rhyme or reason to anything, so it was tempting to think that we made it through not because of some special act or presence of God but because Melanie was young and strong when she got the disease, because she had mental fortitude and toughness, and because she had a caring, loving family and church. All of these circumstances could be viewed as fortuitous. Melanie rolled the lucky dice, and she came out a winner (or, at least, she hasn't come out yet as the loser).

The other extreme, of course, is to think that God was in control of everything the whole time, constantly present, working toward a conclusion divinely sanctioned and ordered. John Calvin once talked about the "hidden bridle of God's providence." Were we, in fact, like horses being ridden around the track, moved by mysterious forces over which we had no control, running not at our own will but at the will of another?

These are, of course, two extremes. Sometimes I think both are right; most often I think the truth lies somewhere in the middle, where it usually lies. The problem is that extreme situations push toward extremes, not the middle. So I try to understand what both images — absolute luck and absolute control — can say and how they can be understood in some less absolute context.

What I have found helpful is Calvin's doctrine of predestination. This may seem surprising to some, but Calvin often used talk of predestination as a pastoral tool to help people in hard situations.

Predestination in this sense — and I think it is the sense not only of Calvin at his best but of Paul — is a doctrine of comfort. Understood from the context of suffering, predestination is just like the Gospel, only maybe more so — it is for the broken, not the whole. As Jesus reminded his audiences, he came for the sick, not the well. The dogma takes a sinister turn only when used by those in power, those not in dire straits, as a doctrinal whip to intimidate.

Calvin certainly knew about brokenness. His own body gave him fits; by the end of his life he was a physical wreck and in almost constant pain. But Calvin also experienced the spiritual brokenness of being exiled from his own country, and he endured the mental anguish of having to deal with those for whom exile was not an option, who ended up at the stake for their religious beliefs, all the while turning to Calvin for counsel. How can you give counsel to those who are being martyred for the faith when you enjoy relative safety? In all these things, we have a key to understanding predestination: it is for those in trouble, in pain, in anguish, because it declares absolutely that God's love is entirely unconditional, which means that none of the horrible circumstances of health or persecution or psychological torment have any bearing whatsoever on our acceptance by God. This predestination is the great affirmation of a "love that wilt not let me go" no matter what. In the final analysis, the notion of predestination can be put to real use only by looking at a Christ who joins in our suffering but is not finally overcome by it; Jesus is raised from the dead in affirmation of God's love despite all that would separate us from it. Predestination, in the end, is not about God's judgment on us but about his love for us. I'm reminded of the lines attributed to Thomas à Kempis: "O love, how broad, how deep, how high; how passing thought and fantasy."

This doesn't mean that predestination — or any religious doctrine — is in any real sense an "answer" to the problem of suffering; there aren't any answers, not of the sort we crave. What it does mean is that we do have a basis, a hope, for continuing to say yes to life and to God; predestination in the sense I have talked about it is a way to begin exploring what life in God's kingdom is like. And, really, it comes down to this point not just for difficult times (for our suffering through this time of cancer, for example) but for the whole of life: when all is said and done, for the really important things there are no answers, only explorations.

And Melanie and I are exploring, exploring several fronts. Of course, there is a devastating illumination that comes at the end of cancer treatment: the end of the treatment isn't the end of anything. Melanie still has to go to the doctor every so often to be checked. She has been declared not "cured" but "in remission," meaning that the leukemia can find its way back and strike out at us again. And it certainly isn't the end of our exploring faith to try to cope with what now seems more real than it did a year ago: the impending possibility of the sudden, quick pop of finitude. That is much more on our minds nowadays, even as the prognosis looks good. We hope, we are happy things have gone well, but we are not deceived.

Another notable person from John Calvin's age, a man named Zwingli, had a close brush with death when the plague swept through his city as it did through many cities during the sixteenth century. In response to his experience, he wrote a poem that is remarkable in the way it maps out the way I as a Christian — and, I think, Melanie — reacted to illness. The poem is divided into three parts, and it seems to me that the essence of each part is captured by its opening lines. "Help, Lord God, help in this trouble," the first part begins. It is a cry to God to do something about the illness, to take it away. "Take out the dart that wounds me," Zwingli cries. And so he joins with Job and countless others through the centuries who have called on God to take care of them in times of trouble.

Of course — and unfortunately for anyone who has had to deal with a tragedy — it almost never works that way. We cry for help, but we do not get help, at least not the kind of help we want: to be miraculously rid of whatever troubles us. Thus, when Zwingli realizes he is sick and will remain sick until the sickness runs its course through his body, his prayer changes: "Console, Lord God, console! The illness grows." The call is now for an assurance of God's presence, not for God's action. Of course, are the two really different? I'm not sure.

The final verse proclaims, "Recovered, Lord God, recovered!" There is obvious joy in those four words. And it is a joy for anyone who has been sick or has gone through an illness with a loved one to be able to say those words: recovered! Yet, this is not a simple or simplistic whoop of joy for a recovery; it is colored by the event of illness itself. In Zwingli's poem, there is within the very verse of praise for recovery a somber realization, much more real to Zwingli after his illness than before, if I had to guess: it is the realization of finitude. He frankly acknowledges in his thanks to God that "I must endure the punishment of death sometime." And so it is. We all know that. Melanie's illness served to underline that fact for our family. Now there is no taking life for granted. We can no longer purchase that luxury; we no longer have the tender of unblemished health by which such naiveté is secured (and secure).

This is one way of saying that life is both beautiful and fragile, full of pleasure and full of pain, all mixed together so that you can't really separate the good from the bad. It's a package deal.

When Melanie was in the hospital the first time, one of the images she used to visualize her fight against cancer was roses: white roses for white blood cells, red roses for red blood cells, and pink roses for platelets. "Let the roses bloom" she would think to herself and tell others. After she had been out of the hospital for a couple of months that first time, we celebrated her birthday (a birthday she spent at home in protective isolation; a friend videotaped the birthday party the church threw for her). I gave her two framed pictures, both portraits of roses by Redoute, one white, the other red and pink. She cried when she opened them. They now hang above our mantle. But now the meaning is a little bit different, at least for me.

Every time I look at those roses, I am reminded of life, of its beauty and fragility. I even allow myself to think in clichés. Life is like a rose: along with the beauty and fragrance and all the other good things, you get the thorns. They are part of that beauty. In a book of essays, Robertson Davies reminds his readers that a saying becomes a cliché when it has a real element of truth in it. So, clichéd as it may sound, I think of life now as a rose.

The pain and pleasure of life have always been intermingled, so entwined with one another as to be inseparable. It's just a bit more apparent to our family now; it intrudes into our thoughts more often.

Our vacation is a good example. A few months after the end of Melanie's treatment, and almost one year after her initial diagnosis of leukemia, we went on a family vacation, traveling from Indianapolis to Washington, D.C., to Virginia Beach, to our home state of Georgia. We were able to travel because Melanie was getting her strength back. It was a wonderful and joyous time, a getting-to-know-you-again time. We spent time with and had fun with the kids; we saw family and friends; we took off sight-seeing and beachcombing. We had fun as we may never have had it before, because we appreciated it more keenly.

But our joy was tempered by our confrontation with death. One vacation day Melanie and I took a drive in the country in my hometown, and we wheeled by the church I had attended as a teenager. It's a little country church that sits in the mountains, a very beautiful place. Melanie began to cry. She had looked at the graveyard and realized that she could die; and if she did, she wanted to be buried in a place where the kids could visit. Before her illness, we had both talked about being cremated in our old age. But now we're not as certain as we once were about reaching old age. And so, as she looked at the graveyard, Melanie thought it was important to think about the kids and their needs. And she was sure they would need a place to visit, a special place set apart, beautiful, to remind them of their mother's life. She hated to think about it that way, but she had to do it. Thinking about death is a part of our life now — not in an overwhelmingly morbid way, but it's there, always, even if it's only in the background.

We both are very much aware now that Melanie may still die. If not from leukemia, then from something. If not now, then certainly later. And not just her, but me, and the kids — and, well, everybody. In a way, it's not that this knowledge of finitude is new; it's just much more real. But more important than knowing that everybody dies is the sense of gratitude for life this experience has evoked. Knowing that Melanie may die (will die eventually) makes me glad she is alive — actively, consciously, aggressively glad. Nowadays I reflect a lot on how glad I am that she's living and remains my dearest companion. More than that, as much as I can, in as many ways as I can, I try to act out my gladness.

This gratitude and this gladness spill over into my Christian life. They shape it. I still have questions, problems, and doubts, just as everyone does. But lying beneath all those things is gladness that Melanie is alive and gratitude that love can be embodied in so real a way that I am able to reach out and touch her. Without this gladness and gratitude, there is no real life. Through this gladness and gratitude, I am able to glimpse a little better what Jesus had a habit of calling the kingdom of God.

This gladness has also spilled over into our sex life. Starting with our vacation, which coincided with Melanie feeling a good deal better, Melanie and I have enjoyed the best and most frequent sexual intimacy of our marriage. For a while, we had intercourse practically every night; now we make love less frequently than that, but still more frequently than before she became ill. We take time for sex, look forward to it, make an effort to share with each other in this way. We pursue sex very intentionally, very vigorously. We're having a great time of it; we enjoy each other's bodies and the togetherness that enjoyment brings in a way that's better than before the illness.

I suppose there's a variety of ways that this could be interpreted. Some psychologists might see it as a grasping after life, or as a need to experience sex as a way of denying death and aging. Others might view it as a frantic attempt to beat away our fears of losing each other. But it doesn't feel that way at all.

For me, anyway, it feels very religious. Sex and the enjoyment of it are an affirmation of life, a nod toward its goodness, a laugh of excitement about being alive. Sex is a good thing, and it's great being together that way, and God is good for making it so. If I understand anything at all about what Father Andrew Greeley is up to, theologically, in his steamy novels, I think this is it. He seems to be exploring the sacrament of sex. Of course, I don't mean "sacrament" in terms of a church ritual but "sacrament" in the older sense of the word, as mystery, a mystery that somehow gives away God's creative presence and work in the world.

At the beginning of this book I wrote about the land of illness as a Babylon. Just because Melanie has successfully completed treatment doesn't mean we've left for the promised land. That still lies in the future. We live our lives in a different place than before the onset of Melanie's illness. We are still traveling through Babylon; maybe we always had been, but we just didn't realize it until the leukemia opened our eyes. But if we are but pilgrims in a strange land, if life on this earth is a type of sitting by the waters of Babylon, then our newfound sex life is, I think, one way that we're learning to sing anew the Lord's song in this strange land.

PART II

THE JOURNEY

I saw a wayworn traveler,
in tattered garments clad,
And struggling up the mountain,
it seemed that he was sad.
His back was laden heavy,
his strength was almost gone,
Yet he shouted as he journeyed,
"Deliverance will come."

— from the gospel song
"Palms of Victory"

CHAPTER XII

The Beginning

Irony: incongruity between the actual result of a sequence of events and the expected results

Melanie died. The second part of this book is about that journey. Here's how it started.

Melanie read the first part of this book when I thought it was also the last part. She sat down and devoured it in one sitting. Then we discussed it a bit, talked about the difference in our perspectives. It was a good experience for us both, for her to have read my feelings and thoughts and for me to hear her reaction. She was warmly encouraging and also helpfully critical. It made us think about what had happened during the past year.

The very next day, Melanie was diagnosed with a relapse of her leukemia. She had called and made the appointment a couple of days earlier. A lingering cold had hold of her. Her arm also hurt; she thought maybe she had stressed it riding an exercise bike, an activity she had picked up within weeks of her last chemotherapy treatment. These were, in a way, small things. But part of her was worried. She actually ended up talking to her oncologist three times before he asked her to come in; he repeatedly told her how unusual it would be for her to relapse so soon after the last phase of her treatment. Just a couple of weeks earlier, all her blood counts had been fine. But for her peace of mind, he said, she should come in.

The next day, I went with Melanie to her oncologist. She had her blood drawn, and he began examining her. Then her blood counts came back. When he looked at the figures, his eyebrows shot up in surprise. We could see the bad news in his reaction. "It's back, isn't it," Melanie stated, without a hint of a question in her voice. Yes, it was back. It had come back. Only four months after her final treatment; only four months after a ten-month struggle of hospital stays, chemotherapy, radiation, and blood transfusions, it was back.

We both cried. I told Melanie that I would take care of her no matter what, that if I spent the rest of my life taking care of her I would count myself blessed. I wish I could have been so blessed, for I now have, I think, much of my life ahead of me, but no one to take care of the way I would have taken care of her.

It was a hard day. We went over the options with the oncologist, though there was only one option, really: start the whole nightmarish process over again or Melanie would die. Another hospital stay would be involved — hopefully only a month or so. Melanie's first experience with induction — ridding the marrow and peripheral blood system of leukemic cells so that healthy cells could grow — had gone smoothly. So we expected it to go smoothly again.

It was Thursday; our older daughter, Mave, was going to start first grade on Monday. Melanie had volunteered to ride the bus, to help children get on the bus that first day and then show them where to go once they got off. She was still determined to do that. So, instead of going to the hospital right away, Melanie, with her doctor's approval, decided to wait until Tuesday to check in. And that's what she did, despite growing pain and weariness.

After we left the oncologist's office, we picked up Mave and Gwynne from day care. It was the day Mave was scheduled to go see her counselor. During the summer, we had started Mave in counseling. She had begun to exhibit certain physical symptoms — primarily a stomachache. After physical causes had been eliminated, Melanie's oncologist gave her the name of a woman who specialized in child psychology and play therapy, particularly in relation to children whose parents had cancer. Mave had been seeing the counselor for about six weeks. That Thursday was to have been her last day. She had successfully processed the stress of the previous year; her complaints of a stomachache had ebbed away. And then came the news, the worst news she could have gotten, as we drove to the counselor's office.

The sound of a child's heart breaking is the saddest sound I have ever heard. Melanie told the girls that she had been to the doctor. Mave's first words were, "But your leukemia won't come back, will it?" And then Melanie had to tell them that, yes, Mommy's leukemia was back. Gwynne, our younger daughter, was really too young to have much of a reaction. But Mave, who was now a six-year-old, responded very differently. She said only two words: "Oh, no." She said them quietly. Then she started sobbing, a sound I had never really heard from a small child. Its soft, inward sound was the sound of a soul crashing in on itself. And I wept for her keenly felt sorrow, a sorrow I would not have imagined a six-year-old child capable of.

The four of us went to the counselor's office and shared our family tragedy and family sadness. And then Mave went to work — working away at her grief, her sense of loss, the feelings of insecurity and fear that dogged her mind's little heels. And we as a family began to work too, hoping for the best, but keeping an eye out for the worst.

Melanie and I always tried to be upbeat yet realistic with the girls. During the past year, we had told them that we hoped the treatment would work, that the doctors and nurses and Mommy and Daddy were working as hard as possible to keep the sickness away. It could come back — that was a possibility — but we hoped it wouldn't.

Now we had been betrayed in that hope.

Melanie did ride the school bus with Mave, but she wished that she hadn't. By Monday she felt very bad. So by Tuesday, her check-in day, she was ready to be in the hospital. We hoped it would be like the last time, that the induction therapy, the initial chemotherapy, would go smoothly and quickly (relatively speaking) — that it would last only a month or so.

We quickly established a routine. Since the hospital was about an hour and a half round-trip from our home, and since Mave was now in first grade, Melanie and I decided that, though I went to the hospital daily, having the girls come every day wouldn't be a good thing. So Tuesdays and Thursdays became "Mommy days" during the week. I would pick the kids up from day care and after-school care in the afternoon, bring them to the hospital, and let them visit with Melanie. Often they would bring pictures they had made, and Melanie would play with them as best she could. After playtime, I would take the girls to dinner in the cafeteria, and then Mave and Gwynne would go back to Melanie's room and curl up next to Melanie on the hospital bed and watch "The Rocky and Bullwinkle Show." Then it would be time to go home.

Both weekend days were "Mommy days," since we spent both Saturday and Sunday afternoons with Melanie. On Saturday morning, Mave would play soccer; on Saturday afternoon, she would tell Melanie all about it when we visited. On Sunday morning, I would preach, since I was filling Melanie's pulpit in her absence; on Sunday afternoon, the kids and I would go to the hospital.

Melanie worked very hard to make the children's hospital visits fun. And most of the time they were. When Melanie was too sick to see them, I would visit alone, without the children. But when they did come, Melanie would have things ready for them. Sometimes she took postcards and drew pictures on them to show the girls all the fun things they would do once Mommy left the hospital. Big "I Love You"'s were plastered all over the cards, and pictures of swings, parks, and zoos spoke of times to come. At other times, Melanie would have stories ready for them. The stories that Melanie wrote in the hospital were beautiful. For Mave, Melanie continued writing the Purple Flower Fairy stories. They always spoke of both struggle and joy, with hope gleaming through the closing sentences. The story called "The Fairy Dance" is like that:

The Fairy Dance

The visit had started out well enough when Mave got to Mommy's room all decked out in the required gown, gloves, and mask. Mommy was in the bathroom after a few minutes. She came out and gave Mave a big hug. Meanwhile, Granny had finally gotten Gwynne into her protective clothing, as well as herself. It was Gwynne's turn first because she was younger and a little cranky from the car ride. So Gwynne sat with Mommy, talking and watching TV while Mave waited somewhat impatiently for it to be her turn. She had brought her new reading book to read to Mommy. It was about a dog named Burton.

Finally, it was Mave's turn, but Mommy had to be in the bathroom again and then again. Mommy listened to Mave read her book, but her stomach hurt her. Soon it was time to go. It was going to be a short visit anyway. Mave went away a little worried. Was Mommy OK? She really didn't get to visit with her very much.

Mave went home. Daddy had to go to the parent night at school and then to the airport to pick up Auntie M and Aunt Margaret. Mave's tummy began to hurt. Daddy explained he wouldn't be gone at night anymore after Granny left. Mommy called to say her tummy felt better. So Mave felt a little better too — but she wished the visit with Mommy had been more enjoyable.

Mave went right to sleep when bedtime came. It had been a long day. She was snoozing soundly under the covers when she began to hear a tiny voice calling her name. "Mave, wake up!" Mave rolled over in her sleep. Surely it couldn't be time for school already. "Mave, get up!" the tiny voice said. "It's me, the purple flower fairy." Instantly, Mave woke and sat up in bed. There was the beautiful fairy hovering before her. The fairy said, "We all wanted to do something special for you. So we thought we would bring you and your Mommy to the full-moon fairy dance." As Mave looked out the window she could see the moon shining brightly in the sky.

The fairy changed Mave's nightgown into a glittering dress, the color of the purple violets that grow in the spring. Then, as they readied themselves to fly out the window, Mave felt the rustling of her wings. They flew deep into the woods. The fairy ring was beautiful, with sparkling lights of all the different flowers hung from the trees. The ring had been cleared of all rocks and branches, and a layer of soft grass had been laid down. Off to the sides were benches for resting and watching, and there was a table full of special fairy treats and fairy punch to drink.

Mave could hardly believe her eyes — then, to add to all the excitement, her Mommy flew down beside her. She looked wonderful in her glittering pink gown, and she even had a pink flower in her hair. She gave Mave a big hug.

Some of the fairies took them aside and showed them how the dances were done. Soon after, the magical fairy music began, and Mommy and Mave were swept up in a swirling and twirling of dancing fairies. Round and round, in and out, parading through chains of fairies with linked arms. Mave and Mommy agreed it was the most fun they had had together in a long time.

After more dancing, Mave and Mommy went over to the treats table. They shared a fairy brownie. Mave chose another delicious cookie, and Mommy got a punch for each of them. Then they sat together on one of the benches, watching the dancing, snuggling together. It wasn't long before Mave felt herself being tucked back into bed and her Mommy whispering "I love you" in her ear.

She woke the next morning right when Daddy called. Ready for school, she walked over to her dresser mirror. She still looked the same — then she saw it. There on her dresser lay the pink flower Mommy had worn in her hair. Mave threw the flower a big kiss and bounded down the stairs, ready for whatever new adventure the day would bring. The End.

Melanie wrote a lot of stories for Mave, but she also wrote stories for Gwynne. Since Gwynne loved dinosaurs, Melanie wrote dinosaur stories for her — like this one:

A Story for Gwynne

Once there was a little girl named Gwynne. She had a big sister named Mave and a Mommy and a Daddy and a cat named Waifer. Gwynne loved to swing and play outside in the park. One day, Gwynne's Mommy had to go to the hospital. Gwynne didn't like it that her Mommy was away. It was hard to play with Mommy on the visits to the hospital; everyone was always saying "Be Still!" or "Don't touch that!"

One night, as Gwynne lay sleeping, she woke up because she heard something scratching at her window. At first she was afraid, and she pulled the covers over her head. But then Waifer the cat jumped on the bed and said, "Gwynne, get up and help me open the window." Gwynne was very surprised; she had never heard Waifer speak before. So she looked out from under the covers. "Waifer?" she said. "Yes, Gwynne," Waifer responded. "Get up, and hurry now." So Gwynne ran over to the window, and she and Waifer opened it.

All of a sudden a big, longneck dinosaur with a happy smiling face stuck his head in the window. "Hi, Gwynne! My name is Charlie. I'm here to take you to your Mom." Gwynne pulled on some pants and a shirt and found her shoes. Soon she was riding down the road, sitting in a basket tied to the top of Charlie's head. Charlie was so big that Gwynne could see over the tops of the trees as they walked along toward the hospital.

Now one of the things Gwynne didn't like about visiting Mommy was that the drive took such a long time. But with Charlie they were there in no time.

And before Gwynne could say "Boo!" Charlie lowered his head and Mommy climbed aboard. All the tubes were gone, and Mommy was wearing her jeans, a T-shirt, and sneakers. She gave Gwynne a big hug, saying, "Aren't we going to have fun!"

Soon Charlie lowered his head again, and Mommy and Gwynne got off at a big park. There were lots of swings and slides and all sorts of climbers. Gwynne and Mommy played and played. After a while they sat down on a bench. Mommy brought out some cookies and milk. They snuggled together for a long time.

The next morning Gwynne woke up in her own bed. She ran to the window, but she didn't see anything unusual. Maybe it was all just a dream. Just then, Waifer came into the room. "Meow, meow," she said like always. Gwynne looked at her, and Waifer winked at her. Gwynne could hardly wait to call Mommy and hear her sing "Good Morning" and talk about their special adventure. The End.

Reality and fantasy, the hard facing of facts and the possibility of hope, are all mixed up in these stories. In this, I think, they are much like the Christian Gospel, if you don't take offense at the idea of the Gospel as fantasy — Grand Fantasy, if you wish, in the sense C. S. Lewis thought of it. The best fantasy enables us to envision the good that is beyond all good, the good that is too good not to be true. I must admit that it has been in Lewis's Narnia stories that Christ has been most real to me — at that very moment when he is most obviously a fantasy figure: this huge lion, "not a tame lion," as it is often said in the books. In fact, it has been the fantastical and its elevating effect on my imagination that have been most useful to me as a Christian. And my family and I were going to need all the fantasy we could get, in the good sense, to help us — if not to stave off the cold, hard facts of reality, at least to put the facts in a frame of reference such that they, and not our spiritual selves, could be tamed.

The hard facts of reality. Almost immediately after Melanie entered the hospital, we were confronted with a choice: whether or not to pursue a bone-marrow transplant. Since Melanie's leukemia was obviously a tougher strain than the doctors had originally thought, they decided that the only real chance for a cure, or even for a reasonable period of remission, lay in the bone-marrow transplant.

We really didn't know very much about such transplants. As I recall, we, along with the larger public, thought they were a real cure, and easily accomplished. But we found out differently. For one thing, the type of bone-marrow transplant Melanie would need required an outside donor. It would be best to have a family member; if that wasn't possible, perhaps someone from the donor registry would do.

But the whole matter of deciding whether or not to proceed became even more complicated when all the particulars were explained to us. We learned that the chances of surviving a transplant for more than a year were not good; they were better with a sibling transplant, worse with one matched from the bone-marrow registry. We also learned that there was such a thing as graft-versus-host disease. The new marrow would be the graft, and the host would be Melanie's body. Basically, graft-versus-host disease means that the white blood cells produced by the new marrow view the host's body as a foreign element, and they attack that host as they would attack a foreign germ back in their original body. The consequences could be devastating: every major organ in the body would be at risk of attack. The most frightening possibility was that the graft could turn against the host's skin, resulting in something very similar to third-degree burns over every square inch of the body. Such a reaction was extremely painful — and always fatal.

The prospects were daunting. Melanie and I seemed to be confronted with a no-win decision: choose death by leukemia, or choose death by bone-marrow transplant. We opted to pursue obtaining a donor, but it was a burdensome choice, and one we weren't sure we would follow through on.

But we began the marrow search. First, Melanie's family was tested to see if any one of them would be a compatible match; siblings were considered to be the best candidates. But none of Melanie's family members matched up with her profile. So we were thrown back on trying to find an outside donor by searching through the registry of bone-marrow donors. This also had the effect of cutting Melanie's already small odds for survival in half.

When we weren't worried about the bone-marrow search, we were worried about whether or not this attempt at induction would work. In order to be a candidate for a bone-marrow transplant, a patient needs to meet certain criteria: the first is that, with Melanie's type of leukemia, a remission has to be induced. That's what Melanie was in the hospital for: a month-long treatment of chemotherapy to rid her body of leukemic cells. The second criterion is good physical condition. Bone-marrow transplants are incredibly stressful on the body, so minimum requirements have to be met in terms of the body's major organs and their state of health.

Once again, as she had the summer before, Melanie made it through her induction therapy, something that couldn't simply be taken for granted: about 15 percent of the time, people don't make it through this stage. Once again, she aggressively pursued her own care, and after about a month she was released from the hospital and came home.

After about five days at home, Melanie had to go to the oncologist's office to get her bone marrow tested, to see if her month-long induction therapy had worked. In this test, the oncologist basically takes a long, strong needle and goes into the hipbone to withdraw a sample of marrow. It is a painful procedure.

I don't think we were prepared for bad news. The first induction attempt had been so easy, and this second time around hadn't seemed to be any different. But the result was different. The leukemic cells were still present in Melanie's marrow. And so, with downcast spirits, Melanie re-entered the hospital. The beginning was over. In medical terms, it had been a failure. And it started a nightmarish middle that neither one of us could have imagined.

CHAPTER XIII

The Middle

(Evil from the Hand of God)

Then his wife said to him, "Do you still hold fast your integrity? Curse God, and die." But he said to her, "You speak as one of the foolish women would speak. Shall we receive good at the hand of God, and shall we not receive evil?"

—Job 2:9-10

"Who is it that urged Job to curse God and die?" Melanie wondered in one of her journal entries. She remembered later on, because she included it in a sermon. It was Job's wife, of course. And, as Melanie's husband, I understood the sentiment exactly: not the part about dying, but certainly the part about cursing God. But even here there is grace, because you don't curse something you care nothing about. "God is good. I cannot not say that. But it must be a terrible kind of good," Melanie wrote. And as I re-read that journal entry, it's so true. Anyone who has been in our situation would want to curse God and die, because that seems so much easier than dealing with the terrible goodness, the goodness that burns away everything and everyone unimportant; the goodness that leaves you relying on no one other than the one you have cursed. C. S. Lewis once spoke of how pain and suffering are the chisel God uses to chip away all that is wrong in us. A terribly good sculptor, that is God, and Melanie became the masterpiece.

Melanie was scheduled for a second round of chemotherapy. It was so soon after the first attempt at induction had failed. Only five days at home and then sent back to the hospital. It hit us like a prison sentence. With a heart weighed down with foreboding, Melanie went back. Once again we were back in the hospital routine, back in the emotional routine, back in the spiritual routine. With a routinized sadness and a routinized faith, we looked forward to the end of this second attempt so that things would finally start going our way again.

Sometimes routine is not at all a bad thing. Adam Dagleish, P. D. James's sleuth, has been well translated to the small screen on PBS's mystery series. At the end of one show, where the killing has taken place in a church, Dagleish sits in a pew talking with a lady whose faith has been shattered by the events, including the death of her priest. He gives this advice, advice given to him by his own priest/father: When your faith ends, keep on acting as if you have faith; when the ritual seems empty, keep performing it.

What's embedded in that advice, I think, is something other than a bow to mere formalism and ritualism. It seems to me that it has to do with the acknowledgment that no human-shaped faith and ritual can withstand the full rigors of life at the point of its most tragic performances. When the mystery of life and death envelops a soul, nothing can withstand the onslaught; so to look to faith and religion as a magic wand that will turn the mystery to banal yet comforting platitudes must, of course, fail. But I do think there is a sense in which the very act of hanging on to faith and religious practice in the face of terror is comforting; neither the mystery nor the pain nor the fear disappears, but the act of hanging on to what is perceived as the good in the face of everything that seems to be contrary to the good is in itself redemptive. Routine in religion, in this sense, is a life jacket that keeps one's head above water until the storms subside, and the soul is once again free to consider the Good that is God.

It was routine that made Job able to withstand the onslaught; and it was routine that sustained Melanie and me. It was routine that helped us, in both cases, to see the Good in the Terribly Good; and it was routine that kept us from being blinded by the Terrible, which would have made us unable to see the Good.

The routine of faith saved us in the struggle. And it was a most awful struggle.

Melanie's second induction attempt also failed, and this carried dire consequences. In order to even be considered a candidate for a bone-marrow transplant, Melanie had to be free of leukemic cells. So, a third induction was planned. It was obvious that the doses of chemotherapy that Melanie had received earlier hadn't been effective; thus, the levels had to be increased. The trick was to get the levels high enough to kill the leukemia without killing Melanie — but they did almost kill her.

Nothing prepared me for how sick Melanie would be. She was so incredibly sick to her stomach that she quit eating. She was fed through her catheter for about four weeks. Her white cells were, of course, wiped out, and everyone knew it would be a matter of several weeks before they would come back — if they came back at all. In the meantime, Melanie was subject to infection. The worst came when a monitoring period was missed because the floor was so busy, and Melanie's vital signs weren't taken for four hours. During that brief time, an infection set in, and Melanie developed an extremely high fever. When it approached 105 degrees, a cooling blanket had to be brought in. Fortunately, the crisis passed.

But then she developed mucousitis. First the inner lining of her digestive tract became inflamed, so she had constant diarrhea despite the fact that she wasn't eating; her body was ejecting burned-off mucous linings. Then the same thing started on the outside of her body, with her extremities. Her hands and feet became beet red, just as if they had been burned. Her doctor started her on morphine to take the edge off the pain. In her fiercely independent way, Melanie continued to care, as best she could, for her own bodily functions. It was heartbreaking to watch her have to get up to go to the portable potty by her bed, intestines fiercely ejecting what little there was inside her. She would hobble the step or two to the seat, her feet a source of intense pain. Yet, she persevered.

Then came the onslaught on her major organs. The most seriously affected were her lungs, heart, and kidneys. The first time Melanie went into congestive heart failure was frightening: she couldn't breathe well; her heart rate zoomed upward, approaching 200 beats per minute; her kidneys didn't eliminate waste the way they should. She was told she would be moved to the next floor up, the floor reserved for bone-marrow transplants and for intensive care for leukemia patients. As the nurses were preparing to move her, she asked me to do one little thing for her: sing me a song, she asked, any song. Melanie liked to hear me sing; I sang to her and the kids, and I sang a lot around the house, with instruments and without. She wanted to hear "Michael, Row Your Boat Ashore." I remember that small request with great sadness because I just couldn't do it. I started the first line: "Michael, row your boat ashore, Alleluia." But I couldn't keep going. Tears welled up inside me, like floodwaters threatening to break through a levee; my body couldn't withstand the fear inside me. I started sobbing uncontrollably, mumbling, "I'm sorry. I'm sorry." Eddies of grief swirled my emotions round and round, sucking me down into the vortex, pulling me into the watery abyss. "I'm sorry." So I laid my head beside hers, and we both cried, I in great heaves, she in shaky, shallow gasps.

Melanie survived. Like a great fighter, she survived. But her heart was malfunctioning, and she became subject to frequent heart failure. Four times in a two-week period she seemed to enter a critical stage. But finally, with the help of a heart specialist, hundreds of pounds of specialized monitoring equipment, and good care, she pulled through, at least in part. Still, the chemo had damaged her heart. We were looking at the prospect — even if by some miracle the chemo worked — that Melanie would be permanently disabled because of her heart.

Once she made it through all of these traumatic experiences and was stabilized again, more troublesome times lay ahead. After four weeks with no sign of a white-cell count of substance, we began to worry a bit. After five weeks, the doctors began to show some real concern. After six weeks, one of Melanie's "substitute" oncologists, one filling in for her permanent oncologist, pretty much said that if the white count hadn't come back by now, it probably wasn't going to come back at all. This meant that it was just a matter of time before Melanie succumbed to some infection or another — a bacteria or a fungus that her body, no matter how much medicine it was given, could not stave off. The fill-in oncologist suggested another check of Melanie's bone marrow to see if leukemic cells were still there, to see if they were the culprits holding down the white count. If the test showed those cells, he said, the most humane thing to do would be to stop treatment and let Melanie die.

At home that night, Melanie's mom and I discussed, for the first time, what to do if Melanie died. It was a surreal experience, calming, much more calming than I would have thought imaginable, talking about where services would be held, where Melanie would be buried. I thought I had resigned myself to her death, and so we started making plans.

The next morning, part of Melanie's family and I sat in the waiting room while the bone-marrow check was done at Melanie's bedside. It seemed to be taking an awfully long time, so finally I wandered back to her room. When I found the door open, I took a step inside. I could hear the oncologist talking to Melanie; the initial diagnosis, he said, was that the marrow was clear. It was clear! I stood by the door a minute; the oncologist seemed intent on continuing to do some work, so I turned and ran back to the waiting room. "It's clear!" I said, over and over again. "It's clear. I thought I was ready, I thought I was ready, but I'm not. It's clear." And for the first time I cried tears of joy in front of Melanie's mom. Before that, I had often refrained from sharing my sorrow, but now I was glad to share my joy. I didn't cry publicly over the bad things; I did cry over this one very good thing. And somehow it made me think that the closest thing to the kingdom of heaven here on earth is crying for joy.

My joy. My joy was Melanie. My joy was that she wouldn't die — at least not today or tomorrow. If the white cells came back, there was still hope. I thought I was ready, the night before and the morning of the test, to hear and accept that Melanie's death was imminent. But I wasn't. And I felt raw joy at the prospect of our life together continuing, at least for a while.

The problem, of course, had not gone away. But since the leukemia wasn't present in the marrow, there was still a chance that the marrow could begin producing blood cells again. The concern was with the white cells, because red blood cells and platelets could be transfused, while white cells, because of their fleeting life span (about four hours), really could not be. So we began our watch for those white cells.

The nurses told us about a little celebration dance they

did when a patient's white cells reached minimum levels again. I told them I would celebrate in advance, that I would do the white-cell dance beforehand, as a way of encouraging the marrow to do its job. Of course, that sounds silly. But it was something I could do. Every morning in the hospital room I did a little dance, assuring Melanie that my "magic" dance would work wonders. And, a week later, it did.

Melanie's bone marrow began to produce white cells at acceptable minimum levels more than seven weeks after the marrow had stopped producing them because of the chemotherapy. All of a sudden, the world seemed better, a good world with a good God. The terrible had passed; the good was upon us. And so we were given hope again.

That didn't mean there wasn't work to be done. The white cells, as well as the other blood cells, did make a comeback. But before Melanie could leave the hospital, her heart in particular had to be stabilized. That became the emphasis. And, after numerous medicinal adjustments by doctors, Melanie's heart was stabilized — not back to normal, but stabilized. The heart specialist told us that, as far as Melanie's heart was concerned, she could live as long as five years in her current condition. That would have been a blessing. But, of course, we weren't focusing on Melanie's heart; we were focusing on her leukemia.

At certain points, language simply fails. What I have tried to do here is summarize ten weeks of intense suffering and pain, but there really is no way to do that; suffering and pain simply exist on their own, outside the realm of language's power to order and control. They have an "is-ness" that defies description, or at least a description that does real justice to the experience.

Maybe that is why it is so hard to express God in our world, and especially God in our suffering, because God has an "is-ness," a simple state of being that makes impossible a description that captures his presence and our experience of it. Yet, God was there in Melanie's suffering, and in my suffering over how to help her in her pain. In a song by a contemporary Christian singer named Wendy Lyre, one of the lines proclaims of God, "My bones are your home." My bones are God's home; Melanie's bones, God's home. Just as pain existed, unmediated by language, so that it was simply a state of almost pure being for Melanie, perhaps that is also how God was present — unmediated by language, at a level of pure being deep within Melanie, inhabiting not just her mind and her heart but her very bones, the source of her leukemic illness and pain. God does not simply comfort us in our suffering; he does not simply offer words of consolation or a spirit of peace, although I think he does those things; God joins us in our pain, and God becomes our pain, taking it into himself and being present to us through it.

In a book called *Theology of Hope,* Jürgen Moltmann discusses a passage from Elie Wiesel's book entitled *Night,* an account of Jewish life under suffering-centered Nazism. Wiesel writes about the young narrator who witnessed the hanging death of some Jewish men, and how he saw God there — God on the gallows, the death of God. But, whereas Wiesel uses this scene to speak of the absence of God, Moltmann reinterprets the story to speak of the presence of God. Moltmann says that God was there on the gallows, that he existed not apart from the suffering and death but within its very midst. Although language failed me, at an existential level within me I grasped Moltmann's meaning, because I had seen it played out in God's bone-level presence with Melanie.

Maybe such a presence can be seen as a deliverance of sorts — a deliverance not from the pain but from the isolation. Having seen this suffering, I know *something* had to empower the hope that Melanie conveyed. Despite her bone-tired weariness, she was uplifted, and I think it had to do with sensing this deliverance. There was no doubt: Melanie was a wayworn traveler, moving through suffering and pain; her flesh was the tattered garment that hung from her being; and life itself was the mountain she climbed. It did seem that she was sad; her strength was almost gone. Yet she shouted deliverance, and God delivered her by joining her struggles, and mine.

Struggling with the bad — the realistic bad, the real bad — by holding to the good; fighting to see being instead of nonbeing even when nonbeing's shadow enveloped the hospital room — these things speak of a deliverance that relies not on rescue but on faith in the good and holding on to the good in the face of suffering. How deep did this go for Melanie? Once again, she played out her own struggles and hopes on the page, when she wrote a fairy story for Mave, one in which she sought to give Mave strength in the face of contrary circumstance. Melanie called the story "The Bad Fairy":

> Once upon a time, there was a six-year-old named Mave. Mave had a Mommy who loved her very much — but Mommy was sick and in the hospital. It was a hard time. Mommy missed Mave, and Mave missed Mommy.
>
> One night, the wonderful purple flower fairy came to Mave's room. Mave had almost forgotten the little fairy who had flown her to see her Mommy.
>
> It happened like this. One night, Mave turned over in her sleep — and suddenly she saw a little purple flower near her bed. She sat up, and as she did the flower bloomed open a little, and a fairy stood before her.
>
> Mave was so excited! "Are you taking me to see Mommy?" she asked. "Will I have wings?" The fairy said, "Yes, you will have wings to fly, but this time we will not see your mother. The good flower fairies need your help. All over the world," the little fairy explained, "there are good fairies that visit children when they are sad and

lonely, and the good fairies help to make hard times a little better. But now there is a bad fairy who has come to our world. He likes to hear children cry, and he feels good when they are sad."

"The little fairies need your help. We need someone to catch this bad fairy with a butterfly net and place him in this jar."

Mave said, "How can I help? I'm just six. Let me call my Daddy."

But the little fairy said, "No. It has to be you because you know us. All the fairies will be helping you to catch the bad fairy, but none of us is able to use the net. So we must have your help."

Very quietly, Mave dressed in jeans and a shirt and socks and sturdy shoes, and then, as she stood ready near the window, the window opened. As she sat on the ledge she heard a rustling sound, and she could see that the little purple flower fairy had given her wings.

And so, with a "1-2-3" Mave flew off the window ledge into the night sky. The fairy took Mave to a place deep in the forest, and there she met all the other flower fairies.

There were flower fairies of every color. Mave flew around admiring all the blues and oranges and yellows and pinks. Mave thought she had never seen a more beautiful sight.

Soon, all the fairies and Mave sat down. The leader fairy began to tell the plan for capturing the bad fairy. The little fairies knew that the bad fairy was making children sad in a town nearby. So their plan was to take Mave there in hopes that they could lure the fairy into a little house there and catch him.

"Mave," the leader fairy said, "you must be very brave, because when the bad fairy comes, he will remind you of sad and unhappy times — he will make you want to cry. Three times he will do this, and each time you must name a happy time. This will make the bad fairy so mad that he will not notice you as you pick up the net. When you have him in the net, then you must spin it around quickly so he cannot escape, and the other fairies will bring the jar to lock him away."

Then all the fairies and Mave flew to a little house on the edge of the town. Once there, they began to dance and sing, to laugh and tell jokes and stories. They made cookies and did some fun projects. They did all these things so the bad fairy would hear and come to the house to make the fun stop.

It worked. It wasn't long before one of the flower fairies guarding the door saw the bad fairy flying toward the house with a mean look on his face. As he came, all the flower fairies hid. Mave continued to play and sing and laugh to herself.

Suddenly, a little brown and moldy-looking fairy came into the room. "Hello," Mave said brightly. "Did you want to play a game with me?"

"Yes," said the bad fairy. "I have a game. It is called the sad game. I will go first, and I get three chances to make you sad. Then it is your turn."

"Okay," said Mave.

Then the fairy said, "I heard that your dog Rapunzel died."

Mave gulped hard and remembered what the purple flower fairy had said about happy thoughts. So she said, "Yes, that was sad. But we got a tree that blooms beautiful flowers in her memory, and I see those and I am happy thinking about Rapunzel. It is a dogwood tree we planted to help us remember how much we loved Rapunzel."

"Hmmph!" said the bad fairy. "Okay. Well, how about

the time your sister got asthma and you couldn't keep your new kitten? How about that?"

"Oh, pish posh," said Mave. "I just go over to my friend Tiffany's house to play with kittens whenever I want. And besides, I love my sister more than a kitten."

"Rats!" said the bad fairy. "All right, I still get one more try. How about your Mom is real sick and is in the hospital?"

A little tear started to form in Mave's eye, and all the little fairies in the room held their breath. Mave thought for a moment, and then she said, "Of course it is a sad time, but I know my Mommy and Daddy love me, and I will be taken care of no matter what. That's what Mommy said. Besides, I will get to visit with her soon, and she is writing me a story."

With that, the bad fairy said, "Well, I can still make you sad. You wait and see." And he flew up and bit Mave on the finger.

"Ouch!" cried Mave, and the little fairy began to laugh in a mean way and roll somersaults in the air. Mave, being very brave, didn't even stop to look at her finger. Instead, she grabbed up the butterfly net and swooped it down on the rolling fairy, then quickly twisted the net so the bad fairy was trapped.

"Hooray!" shouted all the flower fairies as they brought the jar. The bad fairy was quickly whisked away. All the fairies thanked Mave for her help.

The next morning, Mave woke up in her own bed. She sat up, rubbing her eyes. Had it all been only a dream? And then she looked down at her finger. It had a Band-Aid around it. A Band-Aid decorated with all colors of little flowers. THE END.

Was it all worth it? After ten weeks of hellish existence, and with damaged internal organs, Melanie came home. Throughout the story of the bad fairy, Melanie had Mave concentrate on the good and the loving during the sad times. And Melanie herself, with courage and dignity in the face of danger, pain, and indignities, held to the good and the loving — which is another way of saying that she was held bone-deep by the good and the loving, by God. And I believe that it was such tenacious goodness that sustained her, and me, through the battle. And it was with the same tenacious hold on divine love, I believe, that she was able to look at me in bed her first night at home and say, "If I die tomorrow, it's all been worth it to be able to spend this one *good* day at home." The evil from the hand of God had been enveloped, at that moment, by goodness.

CHAPTER XIV

The End

Come unto me, all you who are burdened and heavy laden, and I will give you rest.

— Matthew 11:28

December 1992

Dear Members and Friends
of Danville Presbyterian:

I write you today with hard news. As you know, I have had a long battle fighting leukemia. Throughout this time, you have been very supportive, truly showing the love of Christ to me and to my husband and children.

With sadness I must tell you that my chemotherapy treatments are no longer effective in fighting my disease. After ten weeks in the hospital and as much chemo as one can take, the cancer has returned. I will not return to the hospital for more chemo treatments; instead, my doctor will keep me comfortable as long as possible. We are stressing at this point a good quality of life, not its length. We are looking at a range of a few months to a year, possibly up to two years.

My joys in life are family and church, so I will continue to preach and serve pastorally for as long as I can, with help from Tom. I ask you to continue your prayers for me and my family. Most of all, I ask you to be present with me during this process of living and dying. I am comforted by these verses from Romans 8:37-39: "In all these things we are more than conquerors through him who loved us. For I am sure that neither death, nor life, nor angels, nor principalities, nor things present, nor things to come, nor powers, nor height, nor depth, nor anything else in all creation, will be able to separate us from the love of God in Christ Jesus our Lord."

Much love,
Melanie

Melanie had to prepare this letter less than a month after she had left the hospital. The best thing I can remember about that month is that we went to the symphony. Back in August, once Melanie had relapsed again, I had bought her season tickets to the symphony for her birthday in September. The message was clear: we would not let the leukemia get in the way of our living.

Of course, what happened was that we missed the first performance. In August, during that initial period before we knew what nightmares lay ahead, I had no idea that Melanie wouldn't be out of the hospital in time for an October performance. But she was able to attend the second performance, held in November. It would be the only performance of the six she would attend.

Melanie's mom, the kids, and I had picked out a special symphony dress for Melanie to wear, which we had bought her for her birthday. I have a picture up in my hallway at home, showing Melanie in her symphony dress, a tasteful white turban covering her bald head. I worried that, with her weakened heart, she wouldn't be able to make it up to the nosebleed seats we had, but she did. There she sat, radiant despite the medicine pump and the tubing running into her catheter that carried her much-needed heart medicine. She told me that it was one of the most wonderful days of her life.

And now, a scant three-and-a-half weeks after leaving the hospital, a mere three-and-a-half weeks beyond the torture, she was diagnosed with already having relapsed. The leukemia was back with a vengeance. Again, when she got the news, I was not with her. The first time she had found out about her leukemia, I had taken the children to the doctor; this time, I had my own doctor's appointment. Because she had exhibited no suspicious symptoms, this third relapse caught us totally off guard, and it carried dire consequences.

There would be no bone-marrow transplant. Melanie was too devastated physically for it, and there was really no hope of clearing her marrow with chemo — that had obviously not worked, even in massive amounts.

Again, looking back, I feel very guilty; so often I wasn't there for the diagnosis. This time, when I walked into the house, Melanie was on the phone, sobbing, talking into her sister's answering machine. "It's back" were about her only words.

"It's back." Two small words, yet they shattered my world. We talked about the quality of life and what that would mean medically. Melanie told me that she would be switched to a "palliative" treatment, meaning that now the medicine would no longer hold out the hope of cure but would simply alleviate the symptoms of the leukemia for as long as possible. Melanie had been told that one of her oncologist's patients had lived for two years on this type of treatment. The norm, however, was about four months to a year.

We told the congregation, in the letter above, about the

situation; we called family members; and we sent notes to friends in, of all things, Christmas cards, perhaps a subconscious acknowledgment of how the wonderfully good and the tragically bad are so intertwined in this life. The hardest thing to do, of course, was to tell the children that Melanie would die — not that Mommy might die, not that the treatment might not work, but that Mommy was going to die.

Children who are only three and six have no concept of time, and so it was hard to explain to Gwynne and Mave that Mommy was going to die, but that it would happen in the future sometime. We had to tell them; because of their ages, they had to *not* understand. Mommy was with them now, she was right there in front of them, so how could Mommy die? They were children; I was not a child. Yet the question was the same for me. How could Melanie die? She was right there in front of me. Maybe children aren't the only ones who can't fully grasp time.

Though this should have been the saddest time in our life as a family — the specter of death now so much more substantive, no murky shadows this time but the real thing — it was one of the happiest that I can remember. We had a wonderful holiday season. We spent the time on life, not regrets or fears or questions. And once again, just like the year before, we felt surrounded and supported by the Christmas story, *the* story of life, of a God who got tangled up in human flesh and human life, who lived and died so that people could, at least in the clear moments of life's living, look at death and see life there instead. And that was exactly what was happening with us.

We did a couple of things that, looking back, turned out to be particularly good things to do. One was that we got a video camera. We started taping our life around the house a bit, and we taped Christmas morning. What is interesting is that, on the same two-hour tape that we recorded our joy in Christmas, we also recorded Melanie's last stay in the hospital

— the stark hospital room, the kids visiting, and, finally, Melanie saying good-bye to the children just a few days before she died. And, when I watch the tape now, I see the same thing that I described above: not a woman dying, but a woman living up to the point of her death. There is a difference.

Where does that difference come from, and from what strength? Certainly, the credit goes to Melanie. She chose to take a dark situation and shed light upon it; a hopeless situation became her opportunity to spread hope and good cheer to those around her. Often you hear about people in the final stages of terminal illness who withdraw or who are lonely because people are afraid to be around the dying. But Melanie's aura pulled people in. She opened up herself and others to the good of life. Where others might have seen darkness, she shone forth light, a divine light; she was a conduit for the Good.

Maybe this is why our Christmastime was so good; Melanie's story mirrored in some ways the hope of the Christmas story.

> Watchman, tell us of the night,
> What its signs of promise are.
> Traveler, o'er yon mountain's height,
> See that glory-beaming star!
> Watchman, doth its beauteous ray
> Aught of joy or hope foretell?
> Traveler, yes; it brings the day,
> Promised day of Israel.

So John Bowring wrote in 1825; and now, two thousand years after the "glory-beaming star" shone, it was being reflected in the mirror of Melanie's life. At this point in time, the illness Melanie had suffered through seemed to be the rough cloth that had polished the fragile shell of her life; she was becoming transparent as glass, and the God who had hold of her heart used it to signal to all those who loved her that there was, indeed, a love that would not let go.

And so, this remarkable period of overflowing life continued oh so briefly. On New Year's Eve, Melanie let Mave have a spend-the-night party, even though Mave was just six. I asked her about the sanity of having such a party on New Year's Eve for six-year-olds, particularly when they were promised they could stay up until midnight. Several mothers also raised eyebrows: Do you *really* want to do this, they asked. Yes, Melanie did. Her reason was simple: "I want to do this while I'm still alive." So Mave and her friends, along with her sister Gwynne, managed to stay up till midnight. Melanie made it as much fun as possible for the kids, and when she camped out with them in the downstairs living room, it was with a grin that showed she was really having fun.

About a week later, we had a good snowfall. Framed snapshots on the walls of my house remind me of the best sledding of my life. There are two pictures of Melanie: in one she's standing out in the cold, all bundled up; in the other, she and Gwynne are riding a sled down the hill. Joy beamed from Melanie's face: she was not a sick person sledding; she was a saint sliding across the final few miles of earth's terrain. This was on a Sunday. Melanie had preached that morning; after the sledding we had people over to our house for hot chocolate. The following Tuesday, in the oncologist's office, Melanie told her doctor of her escapades on the snow-drenched hill. "I hope it was gentle sledding," he said with a slight twinkle in his eye, knowing Melanie well enough by this time to have his question answered before it was asked. He knew that she embraced life rather than backed away in fear from it.

The next Sunday night, Melanie and I made love for the last time, on the sofa and floor of our living room. It was long and lusty and passionate. She felt good, smiled heartfelt smiles, and laughed as if there was gladness spilling over inside her.

Just thirty-six hours later, she was back in the hospital. Two days after that, the oncologist told us to call in all the family from out of town, because Melanie probably wouldn't live more than two or three days; they all came. The phrase "crash and burn" was used to describe how quickly events would take place. The phrase startled me when the oncologist used it; the words still shock me now. In a way, they seemed to dehumanize Melanie; they turned her from a person into something like an airplane.

On the Tuesday that Melanie was readmitted to the hospital, a chest X ray had shown an area of infection in her lung about the size of a quarter. Her white cells were no longer up to fighting off bacteria or fungi, so by Friday her lungs were half full of the stuff. The end looked near, and it was, but not as near as the doctor thought.

So many good things happened during what was, in many ways, a dark time. The children came to the hospital often and played with Melanie — as much as she was able to play. Melanie read stories to Gwynne and played hangman with Mave. Some friends from out of town visited; better to see Melanie one last time alive than to come in for the funeral. Friends from church came too; a group of women came to show Melanie carpet samples for the church nursery. The family shared moments with her, mostly talking quietly, laughing now and then, recalling good times. But what was most special was the time she and I spent together, just the two of us. Melanie seemed to be on a high of some sort, fully living out her last days. Though she woke early in the morning, we would stay up until midnight or later each night just talking, and we would enjoy each other's company while she worked on some crewel embroidery pictures for the kids; she was making Gwynne a little girl with flowers, Mave a cat. The hours we spent together were peaceful and quietly joyful.

Once Melanie went to sleep, however, it was a different

story. She would often wake up at night unable to breathe. She received treatments at two, three, and four in the morning. A couple of times I was awakened (I was sleeping in the room with her) by nurses working on her — turning her over, lifting her up, trying to get air into her lungs.. I became so accustomed to this that I assumed that, when Melanie did die, it would be during one of these nighttime attacks. It was a wonder she could breathe at all; whatever it was that was growing in her lungs, one lung seemed entirely full of it, and the other was two-thirds full. We never had the test done that would have told us whether it was a bacteria or a fungus; Melanie's platelet count was so low that the doctor thought she might bleed to death if the test was performed.

In the midst of all this, Mave came down with the chicken pox. She got them from Gwynne, who had had them a few weeks before. This was the very time when Melanie didn't want to be separated from the girls. So, thanks to her gracious oncologist and some very helpful nurses, we arranged to have Melanie transported to a room in a hotel adjacent to the hospital so that she and Mave could visit; Mave obviously couldn't come onto a hospital floor where so many patients had inadequate white-cell counts. Since Melanie was so close to dying, the oncologist didn't think it would matter if Melanie became infected; she would be dead before the incubation period was over, and so she wouldn't be contagious. So, taking Melanie in her wheelchair and carting the oxygen tank, we all met as family in the hotel room, where Melanie was able to touch and hold Mave and Gwynne. The couple of times we did this, it was a great boon to all of us to see mother and children together.

One night, when we were on the way home after a visit to the hotel room, Mave asked why God would let Mommy die. She had tried working it out in all sorts of different ways. I asked her what conclusion she had come to. Finally, she said it was probably so the earth wouldn't get so crowded: if people didn't die, there wouldn't be any room for the new people. Still, she said, it would be better for God to take old people than mommies with children. Then she asked, "Will I remember Mommy?" And the question would have broken Melanie's heart, because that was her question and concern. I told Mave I would help her remember.

The next few days were remarkable. One of the most touching moments came when Melanie thanked her oncologist for all he had done, and then she blessed him. And I truly believe that she did. In fact, she blessed all those around her during those days, especially me. Again, it was this good that brought me to tears, not all that was bad and sad. One morning I awoke about five, and I just sat there and looked at Melanie, remembering our happy conversation of the night before. And then I wept the hardest and longest I had wept during the entire time of her illness. I sat there for an hour, crying, watching her. But the strange thing about it was that my tears were tears of glad acknowledgment, of recognition that, of all the people she had blessed, I had been privileged to be the one she had lavished blessings on the most consistently and faithfully for the past fifteen years. The sadness was there, of course; but it was overwhelmed by the gratitude. Those were good tears to shed.

As it turned out, we had our hopes raised one last time before they were dashed. Melanie should have died by this time, but she hadn't. She had gone to the hospital on a Tuesday; the family had been gathered by Friday. Now it was Wednesday. The lung specialist had an X ray taken, and we discovered that, despite the fact that Melanie had no significant white-cell count, her lungs were much improved. So much so, the lung specialist said, that she could go home. And so, the next day, a Thursday, we packed up and left.

It was exhilarating to be going home. I felt good about it, and Melanie did too. But the first sign of trouble came that night, and from an unexpected quarter. Melanie had her first hallucination. She began seeing things that weren't there, although she was aware that she was disoriented.

I call it the first sign of trouble. This doesn't mean that it troubled me, or that it was medically life-threatening; rather, it was troubling in the sense that the one thing that had scared Melanie the most from early on in her fight with leukemia was that she might lose some of her mental capabilities due to radiation treatment of her brain. This hadn't happened, of course. But those fears had remained, and now they seemed to be realized.

The next day was a Friday. Melanie seemed to have a pretty good day, although she continued to see things, and sometimes she talked in a way that didn't make much sense. But she did make a very cogent comment that was perfectly clear in its implications: "Medicine can keep alive, but it cannot make alive." She had begun to feel her body as a burden, and just because she was being kept alive did not mean that she felt alive. I asked her how she felt about that, and she responded, "There's nothing left to feel. Either I will die or I won't. That's all there is."

When Saturday came, we carried out what seemed at the time a very eerie task: Melanie's mom and I took her to the funeral home to pick out her casket. This is something she insisted on doing for herself. So we loaded up the car, taking Melanie's portable oxygen tank with us, and drove to the home. She had asked me to watch out for her in case she began to talk nonsense or see things, but while she was there the things she said were perfectly clear. She didn't want an expensive casket: she was worried about how much I would have to pay. On the other hand, she *was* the Presbyterian minister in town, and she didn't want her congregation to have to see her in a cheap casket. Finally, she chose a nice blue casket that was medium-priced. And then we left.

By Monday, Melanie was having quite a few hallucinations. She wanted to go back to the hospital because she was feeling uncomfortable at home and, I think, feeling uncomfortable knowing that the girls were bothered by the fact that she often didn't make much sense when she talked to them. At one point, she asked me to look after the white dog behind me. "What dog?" I asked. "You know," she said. "The dog from the agency." "What agency?" I inquired. With an exasperated look, she said, "The dog from the agency for the commercial. Don't you see the three advertising guys on the bench?" I did see, but not what she saw. And that was just another piece of broken heart for me.

Two more days passed. Melanie continued to have hallucinations, but at times she was remarkably lucid. During this period, an old friend from seminary came to say good-bye. Then, on Wednesday night, Melanie said good-bye to the girls. She gave them each a picture of herself, and then she gave them the crewel embroidery pictures she had been working on; one was not quite finished, so a dear friend, Terry, would have to put on the final touches. Finally, she spoke to the girls of being together again in heaven. It was the last time Mave and Gwynne would talk to her, though no one knew it at the time.

Melanie gave me a present too, though she didn't know it. I was working in my study, which is next to the bedroom. Melanie's mom was with her in the bedroom, and they were talking. When Melanie's mom asked her what the happiest day of her life was, Melanie replied without a moment's hesitation, "My wedding day." That is a gift I will cherish for life. Whatever guilty feelings I have experienced since Melanie's death, worrying that maybe I didn't do enough, feeling somehow, insanely, responsible, that gift has sustained me.

The next day, a Thursday, we took Melanie back to the hospital. She was never terribly coherent after that. She really couldn't talk very much. On Friday, her oncologist came by to say a final good-bye and to squeeze Melanie's hand. The chaplain, who had been a wonderful support for Melanie, also came to see her one last time. She did manage to put together some words for him: "This is a weird experience," she said, and smiled. These experiences were relayed to me by Melanie's mom; I wasn't there. I was resting a bit; I was sick myself.

I did go in and spend the afternoon with her, mostly watching her as she rested, and then I went home to tend to the girls. I talked to Melanie on the phone about 8:00 p.m. She managed to say "I love you" and "Goodnight." I could understand her, though her words were very slurred. Her mom told me that they had been singing hymns — at least, Carolyn had been singing while Melanie hummed along.

About 10:00 p.m. I got a call from the hospital. Melanie had taken a turn for the worse; her breathing was terribly labored. So I made my way back to the hospital quickly (or at least as quickly as one can make a drive that takes 45 minutes). My father was there, as were Melanie's mother, stepfather, and father. Melanie never really seemed to regain consciousness; we just heard grunts occasionally. I sat up with Melanie, dozing part of the time, until 5:30 a.m. Finally I left her room and slept in the visitors' lounge for a couple of hours; then I went home to shower, change clothes, and rest a bit.

I was called back about noon on Saturday, and I was at the hospital by one o'clock. Melanie was remarkably worse. I say "remarkably" because I couldn't have imagined anything worse than the night before. Her breaths now came in great gasps; she was locked in a fierce struggle. It was such a hard struggle that I think her body had to rest in between breaths. For the next hour and fifteen minutes I expected every breath to be her last, since such a long time elapsed between breaths.

Melanie's eyes wouldn't close; they were about half open. Tears occasionally ran from her eyes — ostensibly because, since her head was turned and her eyes weren't closing, the tears, rather than being distributed by blinking, gathered at the corners of her eyes and ran down her cheeks. Her nose also ran a little bit. The nurses, along with my dad, assured me that she wasn't really conscious. Still, I sat there, wiping the tears from her face, thinking it looked too much like crying. Bubbles under her skin, like blisters, had formed on her nose. Every so often I would lean over and whisper in her ear, "I love you, and Mave and Gwynne love you."

Melanie's folks went for lunch soon after I got there. They came back about 2:00 p.m. At 2:15 on Saturday, February 6, 1993, Melanie died.

That was a shock for me. I had always expected Melanie to die at night, not during the daytime, with the sun shining, with light drenching the room. For some reason, I had expected death to come under cover of night, an unwanted visitor who had to slink in unawares and snatch what I didn't want to give up. Death seemed all the more wrong for coming in the sunshine.

It seemed to me that there was a shocked look on Melanie's face. Right at the end, she gave two big moans and a gasp. And that was it. I leaned over and again whispered, "I love you and the kids love you." Then I said, "Go in peace, friend." She was the best friend I ever had.

We called the nurse in; she said Melanie's heart hadn't quit beating quite yet. But, within a matter of minutes, it had. Then the ritual of "official" death began. A doctor was called in to verify Melanie's state and sign the death certificate; the chaplain came in to say prayers. The nurse began to "unplug" Melanie. After the doctor signed the death certificate, Melanie was taken away. We packed up Melanie's few belongings, and we all went home. This was hard, but something harder still faced me.

After confirming the arrangements we had already made with the funeral home, I had to make phone calls, and that was a surreal experience; I had never had to call anyone before and say "My wife has died." That may sound like a bad joke, but I mean it. To have to say something like that when there has been absolutely nothing in life that has prepared you for it is disorienting at best. You don't know how to say it, how much emotion to let out, how much information to provide, how much comfort to give and how much to receive. It was a totally alien and alienating experience. Such little words — "She has died" — for such a big experience. Language is, at times, a cage.

The hardest part came when it was time to tell the children. After I finished making the phone calls, a friend who had been keeping Mave and Gwynne brought them home. I took them up to the bedroom Melanie and I had shared. Almost immediately Mave asked, "Is Mommy dead yet?" It was a question she had started to ask every time I had come home from the hospital for the last few weeks. Melanie and I had told her that Mommy would die. She just wanted to know when it happened. And, up until this moment, I could always look at her reassuringly, give her a big hug, and say, "No, sweetheart, Mommy hasn't died yet." And then she would heave a big sigh of relief. A ritual had developed, and Mave had begun to feel comfortable asking the question, because she was comfortable with me saying no.

But this time I couldn't say what she wanted to hear. "Yes," I said. "Yes, Mommy has died." A terrified look of shock passed over Mave's face, and she started crying. Gwynne, though she wasn't old enough to take it all in, felt the emotional sadness sweep over her sister and joined her in crying. And I felt so bad because it seemed I was always the bearer of bad news: Mommy is sick; Yes, Mommy is getting better; No, Mommy has had a thing called a relapse; Yes, the medicine is working; No, the medicine is not working; Yes, Mommy gets to come home from the hospital; No, Mommy is not better and has to go back to the hospital; Yes, Mommy is still alive; No, Mommy has died. There it all is: a record of false hopes and promises, stricken with the marks of ugly reality, the unmaking of the good reality they had known as "Mommy." And I felt responsible; I was the one who constantly destroyed their worlds. For that, and for so many other reasons, we cried together.

The visitation at the funeral home, which was held on Monday, two days after Melanie's death, called forth the best of people and the best in people. Friends, parishioners, colleagues — all the folks who had journeyed with Melanie the wayworn traveler came to pay their last respects. And though all were sad, many managed both a smile and a laugh, as we all tried to remember the good and beautiful and true that had been Melanie. And those memories, even in the midst of death and a funeral home, at times brought forth laughter that was like a balm to the ragged red scourge lines running along my emotional back.

Melanie herself had planned the funeral service, which was held at her church on Tuesday. Ironically, she had written her Doctor of Ministry paper on funerals. In her service she had tried to put her theory and beliefs into practice, and it showed. It was a lovely service; sad, yes, but with a current of joy, love, and hope running beneath it all and, at times, overflowing. It was a fitting witness to the Christian doctrine of resurrection.

All the family members made their way to Georgia for the burial; Melanie would be laid to rest in her hometown of Carrollton, Georgia. This time the funeral visitation was more draining for me — there were so many people I didn't know. And the atmosphere was more melancholy than it had been back in Indiana.

Melanie had died the Saturday before; the burial took place on a Friday. There was a brief graveside service; I was the presiding minister. And, with words too inadequate to repeat here, words inadequate to measure either the sorrow or the hope, Melanie Ann Lane was laid to rest.

"Come unto me, all you who are burdened and heavy laden, and I will give you rest," Jesus said. Melanie's burdens were now laid to rest: gone were the pain and the suffering, the dashed hopes and despair; gone was the alienating world of sickness, where tubes made unwelcome inroads and invaded the body's privacy; cast aside was the body that had turned against its owner in a cruel and often mocking manner — all of that, cast aside with the body at the grave.

The Christian hope is that, after the nonessentials are cast out, burned away, put aside, it is the essentials that remain, dear to God and preserved by God. Love and joy — everything in Melanie that was love and joy, I have no doubt, remains. Love and joy: these are Melanie at her purest, that which God had refined by the fires of earthly existence, and which he keeps, now and forevermore. That is the Christian hope, and mine. Melanie's love and joy become clearer to me each day; that is her legacy to me, and God's promise to us all. And therein I find that my own burdens, burdens that so often make life seem so heavy laden, are put to rest; in, through, and by the power of him who showed forth most clearly these promises of God, Jesus my Lord.

CHAPTER XV

Keeper of the Nail Clippings

(The Sickness unto Death)

When death is the greatest danger, one hopes for life; but when one becomes acquainted with an even more dreadful danger, one hopes for death. So, when the danger is so great that death has become one's hope, despair is the disconsolateness of not being able to die. . . . [If] for a single instant this experience is possible, it is tantamount to experiencing it forever.

— Søren Kierkegaard

Through me is the way into the doleful city; through me the way into the eternal pain, through me the way among the people lost. . . . All hope abandon, ye who enter here!

— Dante's *Inferno*

December 6, 1993

Dear Abbie,

I was glad to get your letter today. Melanie died ten months ago today. It's been a hard day. I still relive February 6 every day. I see her struggling for breath; her eyes won't shut, so tears form and roll down her cheeks, and I wipe them. Everyone says, "She isn't conscious, so she isn't in pain." But with her eyes open and tears coming out — it's the image I live with. I keep wondering if I should have done something different, but I don't know what that would have been. I try to remember the good, beautiful, and true. I go back to a poem I wrote for her:

A beautiful spirit danced my way,
  it was just the other day.
Yet years it seems that I have known,
  the grace and joy that she has shown.
An elegant spirit, this one seems,
  all laughing eyes — glad sunbeams!
Her bearing regal as a rose,
  with a grace and a beauty all her own.

The rose has faded; only thorns remain — they pierce my heart! The pain is winning today. I don't know if I will actually mail this — it must be depressing to read. I will respond to your letter in a few days. But, tonight, I needed to write this. Thank you, Abbie, for your friendship.

This letter, which I did send, indicates both the despair and the grace that have come my way since Melanie's death. The despair, I think, is obvious. What is not obvious is that I wrote this letter to a friend from many years before who had reached out to me from over 600 miles away to be a support to me;

so, while I speak explicitly of despair, there is also in this letter the grace of friendship that supports so much of my life in this period. These two things — grace and despair — dominate my life now, are clear to me. I will deal with grace in the next chapter; in this one I will try to explain the despair.

Kierkegaard is right; when you're in the midst of despair, it is not for a minute, or an hour, or a day — it's forever, existentially. In other words, at the moment you are gripped by the forces of despair, you simply cannot imagine that the despair will ever end, which simply reinforces the power of the despair. It does have an eternal quality; it gives you the feeling that hope has been abandoned for life in the eternally doleful city. It is not that, while you are in the despairing moment, time stands still; time is irrelevant to the experience.

How can this despair be described? Language again falls short. There is pain, hurt, humiliation, loss of self-esteem, and a bone-wearying sadness — all of that is in despair. But if I had to pick one word that comes closest to describing how those feelings are experienced, I would have to say "dull." The deadening dullness of despair is what overwhelms me into an existential eternity of sickness unto death. Each moment that is grasped by despair is so incredibly dull that there seems to be no end to the dullness; it makes my existence dry, colorless, and joyless. Having characterized this state with one word, I have to go on to say that there are not enough dull words in the English language to be able to convey how dullness sometimes soaks completely into every fiber of my being. It is a sickness; it is a living death that sucks the good out of life.

No words. As a teacher, I make my living with words; as a minister, I proclaim the power of words, The Word, to overcome. Yet there are no words to express the dullness that I feel. Even sadness loses its acuity; what I feel is a dull kind of sad.

I've tried to express the way I feel, but I can't. I told a counselor that the only language appropriate to these feelings is the language of death. At times it seems clear to me that the only way to truly express the pain I feel at Melanie's death is to die — to commit suicide. How can one truly express the pain involved in the death of a loved one except to die? But I wouldn't do that — Mave and Gwynne need me too much. And again, there is the problem. To say "I want to kill myself" doesn't seem to carry the force of the words unless you actually follow through; otherwise, it can be seen as an act of melodrama. In any case, communication of feeling is barred by the inadequacy of the language.

I once put a knife to my chest and pressed in, just to see how it felt. I wasn't suicidal. But I did want to focus on the possibility of death as a release, death as an answer to questions, death as a reunion with Melanie. Yet I knew I couldn't die now; and, as Kierkegaard knew, that was in many ways the source of my despair. I would simply have to continue my dull existence.

In this type of despairing dullness there is a boredom, but not a boredom that comes from there being nothing to do. In fact, I have plenty to do, much to keep me busy, constant claims on my attention. But, because I am in despair, I mechanically go through the motions of busyness, and things hold no interest for me in any meaningful sense. And there's the rub. There's a Peanuts cartoon in which Charlie Brown asks Lucy how life is going. Lucy replies with a long list of things she has accomplished. Charlie Brown then asks, "Yes, but what does it all mean?" To which Lucy retorts, "Mean? Mean? I thought the point was just to stay busy."

I am busy, but despair drives out the meaning. I think this explains the contradictoriness of the following two things: (a) most people who know me have remarked on how well I seem to be doing, based, I think, on the fact that I have continued to fulfill my responsibilities and to do so very well; and (b) I almost resent being told how well I'm doing, because being told that seems to pass over the fact that I *don't* feel I'm doing anything well and that there can be no sense of well-ness ever again. How do you "handle well" the death of that which is dearest to you? For people to suggest that I can simply move past that loss and do well — that comes almost as a slap in the face of how I actually feel about things.

But, as I said, I think this state of affairs is explained by my feeling of despair and the way it robs me of meaning in my daily activities. Everything I do, the things I accomplish, the tasks well done — all remain very much external to me; they are not a part of me because the very thing that would make them a part of me, meaning, is the very thing that has been suffocated by the weight of despair.

It isn't just that you feel distanced and disconnected from things; when you are gripped by despair, you feel distanced and disconnected from people. What despair does most to you is leave you to yourself. There is nothing else — only you and your despair. No God, no spouse, no friends; despair is isolating. You are completely your own, and that is a terrible feeling to have. It is hell, as George Macdonald knew. At nighttime, when the dark loneliness descends, it is the worst. So I sit up late at night, dog tired yet afraid to go to bed to lie with the loneliness that waits for me there in its black, entangling, web-like nightgown. Middle-of-the-night talk shows about lesbian-nun-lovers-who-have-had-sex-change-operations-while-shut-up-with-aliens-so-they-could-go-back-in-time-and-father-their-own-mothers seem welcome company in the face of such despairing loneliness. And that is sad. And it is hell. Martin Luther knew what he was talking about when, in his Ninety-Five Theses, he equated despair and hell. These late nights are my domain of anguish, where I and I alone exist — a domain, to use a phrase from friend and scholar Kyle Pasewark, "barren, empty of hope, a theatre of despair." Night after night, I am on stage.

The problem is sometimes exacerbated by the pictures of Melanie's absence. Can you have a picture of a thing absent? I think so. My whole house is a portrait of her not being here. It seems that everywhere I look, everything in my house is a snapshot of her not being here. I see the pictures on the wall: the two framed prints of roses, a birthday present for Melanie; one of an English country home, a Christmas present. I see the wooden sculptures from the Philippines, a madonna figure and a pied-piper figure, given to her as gifts. I sit on a sofa she picked out six weeks before she died; at the store she had laughed and said, "I hope I live to see it delivered." It doesn't seem too funny now. I hold a flute she gave me, her last Christmas present for me. It had to be back ordered. Not only did it not come before Christmas; it didn't come before she died.

Then there was the application for a grant for my academic research, which still occupies much of my professional life now. When Melanie read the grant application a little more than a month before she died, a tear ran down her face. When I asked her why she was crying, she replied, "Because I won't live to see all the things you'll do and write." The letter indicating that I had received the grant was on my office desk, waiting for me, the first day I went back to work after her funeral.

Everywhere I look, I see pictures of the missing Melanie. It's most obvious when I look at the children. When I feel inadequate to the task of raising them without Melanie's help, when I look into their eyes and see my shortcomings as a parent, that is when the portrait of Melanie's absence is most clear to me.

Of course, in their own childlike way, Mave and Gwynne mirror their own despair over the loss of their mother. They know what it means now to have a broken heart, to live with distrust of the world, to sorely miss the love of their lives. Sometimes they sit together at night, holding a picture of

Melanie, crying their little hearts out. And with their sadness come other concerns. Both Mave and Gwynne have asked me if I'm going to die too. And when I try to reassure them that I won't die for a very long time, I think they can only half believe me.

Mave's concerns have come out in other ways, too. One night shortly after Melanie died, I found her crying. "What's the matter?" I asked. "I'm the only one in my class without a Mommy," came her reply. She felt separated, isolated from her classmates by her grief. She was in first grade when Melanie died. It seemed to me tragic that, once spelling had become a subject, she wanted to be sure she could spell "die" correctly. "How do you spell 'die'?" she had asked me one night. And then she had written it out for herself, over and over, trying to fathom not just the letters but also the meaning.

And she is old enough — so young, but old enough — to understand my grief. Shortly after Melanie died, Mave and I were riding down the road and listening to a cassette tape by the Chieftains, an Irish band, playing with the singer Van Morrison. In one of my favorite songs, there's the line "She's the wee lass who's left my heart broken." When she heard that, Mave looked up at me and said very matter-of-factly, "I know who's left your heart broken. Mommy."

Gwynne, who is three years younger than Mave, has had to start working through her grief in a different way. Early on she expressed concern about Melanie's welfare. Typical questions were ones like, "Where's Mommy's pillow? What does she sleep on in heaven?" She also seemed concerned with the physical process of death. Not long after Melanie died, Gwynne began to ask, "Has Mommy turned into bones yet?" For several weeks I answered "No, probably not," though I didn't feel compelled to call anyone to try to find out when an embalmed corpse actually did start to turn into bones. But as it turned out, Gwynne was after a different kind of information. I learned that the day I responded to her usual question with the usual "No, probably not," and she asked, "Well, then, can we go and dig her back up? I miss Mommy." And she began to cry. And so began the process of her understanding what being dead means. She asked her questions not to get facts; she wanted her Mommy back.

She also began to ask if she could wear Mommy's clothes when she got bigger. At first I thought this was a way of indicating that she wanted to be close to Melanie. But then she began to talk about sharing the clothes with Mommy if Mommy ever came back. And that was when I realized that Gwynne wanted not only a closeness but also a sharing that had less to do with Melanie's clothes than with Melanie herself. She wanted her Mommy, and this was one way she had of telling me that.

The fight, of course, is with time and blurred memories. What despair threatens to do at its worst, I think, is to overwhelm the children and me both by turning Melanie's physical absence into the overriding psychological factor in our lives. Melanie's beautiful memory, the good that she was, the good that she was that continues to live in the children, in me, in her family and friends — all of that is what is important to remember. And the theatre of despair is the stage on which those good things are threatened with extinction, because the dullness of despair, over time, blurs the good memories so it seems only the bad ones survive. This is what is tied up, in part, in Mave's too-old-for-her-age statement that she made just the other night. With tears in her eyes, she proclaimed, "It's hard living on the edge."

For what, finally, are we left with? One day when Melanie was in the hospital, she was clipping her toenails, and I gathered up the clippings to throw in the trash can. It became a joke of sorts; I was given the official position "Keeper of the nail clippings." Yet, in the quagmire of despair, it is no longer a joke; sometimes it seems to me that this is the role in life I have been given — I have been left with the dry, hard, lifeless clippings to hold, and nothing else. And if that were truly all I had left, then in fact I would be living a sickness unto death, always, eternally, standing under Dante's inscription. And there would be no deliverance for this wayworn traveler.

These are the times of my unfaith. Paul warned the Thessalonians, "Don't be as the pagans, without hope." Yet that is the password to the doleful city: without hope. And when I am in that city, I am a pagan, and I feel like one.

CHAPTER XVI

The Lark Ascends

For all the saints who from their labors rest,
Who Thee, by Faith, before the world confessed,
Thy Name, O Jesus, be forever blest:
Alleluia, Alleluia.

— From "For All the Saints," words by William Walsham How, tune by Ralph Vaughan Williams

"Mirror of Joy"

Psalm 137:1-4;
1 Thessalonians 5:16-18

Dear Friends,

I want to say this morning that this sermon is about Melanie — about how I feel about things, and how my faith relates to issues surrounding her sickness and death. I will not make this a habit — Melanie would not want me to. But it seems unnatural, standing here in her pulpit, her place, only a week and a half after her death, not to have at least one sermon that acknowledges her loss and how I understand it. And so, that is what I do today.

I loved Melanie with a special love — perhaps all people who truly love each other feel that way. But that feeling of special love was reinforced by other people's observations. When I called my best friend from graduate school to tell him of Melanie's passing on, his first sentence was "You two were so much in love." This coming from a person who didn't know us until we had already been married six years, long enough for the newlywed part of love to have faded. Yet, what remained was stronger, better, purer — and it showed to others.

It is ironic that the way I have always thought of our love was captured in the first two stanzas of Edgar Allan Poe's "Annabel Lee." Perhaps you know it.

> It was many and many a year ago,
> In a kingdom by the sea,
> That a maiden there lived whom you may know
> By the name of Annabel Lee.
> And this maiden she lived with no other thought
> than to love and be loved by me.
>
> *She* was a child and *I* was a child,
> In this kingdom by the sea.
> But we loved with a love that was more than love —
> I and my Annabel Lee —
> With a love that the winged seraphs of Heaven
> Coveted her and me.

Sometimes, just as in the poem, I feel that we were children when we married — I was nineteen. Yet it was no child's love. What a marvelous line: "We loved with a love that was more than love" — Melanie taught me what that meant, how it could be true. Of course, I said it was ironic that I liked the poem and saw our marriage through its words — "loved with a love that was more than love" — because, of course, in Poe's poem, Annabel Lee dies young.

How does one go about describing a love that is more than love? What does it mean to feel that way about another person? How are two people to be seen who feel that way? I've always thought it's like two people being a part of the same song. Our life together, Melanie's and mine, was music. I tried once to capture this feeling in a poem I wrote for her, "Variation on a Wedding Theme":

Notes fall from starry clefs,
  through time into time,
Cacophonous at first,
  but then melodies of people emerge
    from heaven's strains.

And music walks incarnate —
  in human form.
A symphony of strength, love, and compassion,
  gentle pianissimos mixed with
The violent upheavals of emotional fortissimos.

Quietly, a fugue unfolds,
  subtle, yet distinct.
Melody chasing melody until,
  caught and entwined,
The Two become one.

We are the music,
  and you are my love.

"We are the music" — that was Melanie and me. And now, part of the song is gone. The music that enraptured my life has passed on to the heavenly chorus.

This feeling, and the dreadful fears of the last year and a half, are why I return again and again to the question of the Psalmist: "By the waters of Babylon, there we sat down and wept, when we remembered Zion. . . . How shall we sing the Lord's song in a strange land?" How to sing? How to sing when dragged down from the land of bliss and normalcy, a life that had a future, into a land of strange medicines, tubes, and pumps, a land foreign to all hopes and dreams of a life together. Melanie and I did more than sing the Lord's song — we felt we *were* the Lord's song, our lives the music of praise, as we faced life together. Yet, how to sing in the land of exile? That was our question. And now, more so for me, I sing alone — Can I be music for the Lord without my accompaniment? It truly has felt, and does feel, like an exile to a place I do not want to be, yet must walk, and walk alone.

If you want to know what it feels like — though many of you already do — it's like walking in a deserted, dark place. One of the lines from Psalm 23 — "the valley of the shadow of death" — can be translated to read instead "the valley of deep darkness." I walk now in a valley of deep darkness. It's like being in the mountains, down in a narrow ravine, between two high, steep ridges. A place always dusky, always moist — the sun does not shine: sides too steep, trees too tall. And once the sun goes down, the duskiness changes to darkness. And you must walk in that valley of deep darkness, reaching in front of you, touching moss-covered trees with outstretched hands, always in danger of running into unseen objects — trees and rocks — hoping to find your way. Groping, groping for a path that leads you out into the light.

That seems a desperate situation, and sometimes it feels like one. But imagine the lost soul's joy [upon] hearing a stream — a stream — a pathway of water that will lead out of the deep darkness. A sure direction to follow; water to drink; a welcome sound — the rushing of water leading outward, forward, away.

Thank God that in my valley of deep darkness I have a stream to follow — it is the living water of God's Word. A fount of nourishment, a place of refreshment as I walk through and out of the deep darkness. God's Word — that which carries one into the light of day, a deliverance from the shadows of doubt, should-have-beens, and tormentful self-questioning.

It is that source which has fed my faith. And especially it has been that saying of Paul's: Rejoice in the Lord always. Rejoice in the Lord *always*. It refocuses my mind, makes me think what it is I should be joyful about, what should fill me with contentment, even in these times. To rejoice in the Lord is not to deny that there are valleys of deep darkness that we must all walk through, but it is to affirm that we do not walk alone. Rejoice — in the face of Melanie's death. How do I rejoice? Paul makes me think about that, and I am glad he does.

Glad because I am thankful — there are things of joy to know even now. Most of all, I am glad that God loves me, and that God loves Melanie. *God* loves. Think of that — the Creator, Sustainer, and Redeemer loves us. The one who creates galaxies with a word, showers light with a thought, forms worlds at will — that God loves us, loves me, loves Melanie. The power of the universe that makes all things alive through his breath cares for us. If such a God loves us, what do we have to fear? "O love that wilt not let me go," the old hymn says. A love that will not let go. A love that in all circumstances holds us to himself. That is joy, friends, to have a glimpse of and a longing for such as that.

This is not an act of denial — oh, there is still sadness. I once told someone that what I felt was a dry kind of sadness — a desert sadness, where each grain of sand is an unshed tear. There's no denying that. But joy comes from realizing that beneath the sands of sadness is a foundation, a rock, that upholds us in our sadness, that is firm in support, that will not let us sink. And that rock is the God who keeps each of us for his own. That is joy — not denying the sadness, but knowing there's something deeper and better and stronger which we desire and for which we hope — the love of God. That is joy, even in times such as these.

How do I know this? How can I trust it? Because I have seen the face of God that makes joyful the downtrodden. I have seen the face of God. Where? Let me tell you something. John Calvin once said that there are things in our world that serve as mirrors of God. Mirrors of God. Things that reflect for us God's love, beauty, truth, and joy. I have looked into one of these earthly mirrors and seen the goodness of God.

I have seen God reflected in Melanie's eyes. Oh, I used to study those eyes. And there I saw compassion and strength, love and mercy, kindness and gentleness. And there I saw joy — the joy that comes from a loving heart, knowing it is kept in the hands of God. Melanie was, for me and for many who knew her, a mirror of God. And, as such, she was a mirror of joy.

So, I can rejoice in the Lord; I know to trust his promises; I can relax in his care; I can faithfully hold to his rod and staff. I can do this because I have lived with and loved a woman who was a mirror of joy indeed.

And so, God bless her; and God bless me; and God bless you. Rejoice in the Lord always; again, I say, rejoice. Amen.

In an earlier chapter, I related a sermon I preached early on in Melanie's illness, a sermon full of hope, and then I talked about wanting someone to come up afterward and ask me if I believed it. To some extent, I felt hypocritical about proclaiming so boldly something I could not fully bring myself to believe. One could also ask the same question about this sermon, I suppose, but in many ways it no longer seems to me as important a question as it did earlier. I think the explanation for that is simple: my life is much more attuned to the paradox, the ambiguity of life, since Melanie died. In my heart, I know much more about the interweaving of despair and hope. So, in a sense, there cannot be one answer; it is, and always will be, two answers: yes and no. Yes, I do believe the hope I preached here. No, I do not believe it. How do I explain this?

"Lord, I believe; help my unbelief," someone once said to Jesus. I now think that this state of belief and unbelief, of assurance and despairing doubt, is normal. It just takes something as devastating as the death of the one you love dearly to bring clearly to consciousness this state of mind.

Jesus knew it, and the Psalmist knew it. "My God, my God, why have you forsaken me?" both ask. And now, to illustrate my point, I'm going to take a longish look at a few quotations from John Calvin, the person I spend much of my professional life studying. Thus far I have refrained from any long discussions about Calvin's theology because I knew it would turn this book into something too much like a dissertation and less like what I wanted it to be: an exploration of my spiritual state throughout Melanie's illness and death. And yet, Calvin has been with me all along; he's all between the lines if you know where to look. But, on the point at hand — belief and unbelief, assurance and doubt — he's just too good to pass up.

Psalm 22:2 is the verse that follows the Psalmist's cry of abandonment: "O my God, I cry by day, but thou dost not answer; and by night, but find no rest." Calvin says that this situation "is what every one of the faithful experiences in himself daily, for according to the carnal sense he thinks himself forsaken by God while yet he apprehends by faith the grace of

God." Forsaken yet assured; despairing yet faithful. That's just the way we are, and to demand absolute belief in a sermon such as mine is simply impossible. We are too frail for that; our intellect is too small to ultimately rationalize the mysteries of living and dying. That's why, with Calvin, pure intellectual assent, what often passes for "belief" when people use the word these days, is unacceptable. He knows the gospel is too big to be contained by the cranium. That's why he insists that the true knowledge of Christ, in terms of belief, of doctrine, "is a doctrine not of the tongue but of life. It is not apprehended by the understanding and memory alone, as other disciplines are, but it is received only when it possesses the whole soul, and finds a seat and resting place in the inmost affection of the heart." There is a logic to Calvin's thought, but it is, as one scholar has noted, a "logic of life, of reality."

A logic of life; I like that. A logic which states that I can be in the depths of despair, and yet, YET, that there's a part of me, my inmost heart, where I can receive Christ and be comforted. And this comfort comes not from the despair disappearing, as though the pain were unreal and the dullness an illusion. It comes in the very midst of the despair, as a spiritual insight; my heart is gripped by a power that causes me to sit up and take notice of the grace that surrounds me. And the best I can do to describe this experience is to say that it is a feeling of the goodness of life; there are moments when darkness is pierced and light shines into the soul. And it is irrelevant, almost, to ask if I believe it, as one would believe the logic of a syllogism. A wise and generally underappreciated man from the sixteenth century, a man named Erasmus, once said, "The philosophy of Christ is not a matter of syllogism but of feeling." In other words, Christianity is more a matter of affection, of feeling, than of strict reason — a matter of having a heightened sense of awareness; of understanding feeling as a sense of the interior of the soul rather than as simply emotion; of being able, amid the rubble of a destroyed interior life, to imagine a good, the good, Goodness itself. And the proper response to such Goodness is not to analyze it, not to syllogize it, but to simply proclaim it. And in the proclamation of it, there is the hearing of it; and in the hearing of it, there is the imagining of it; and in the imagining of it, there is a transformation whereby the heart is taken outside of itself and reformed, recreated by God himself, so that it is a heart more and more able to take in the good. And finally, through the wonderful act of proclamation and imagination, God works to make us new creatures. Not in spite of the despair that I know, and all the world finally comes to know at one point or another, but through it.

Life's meaning, then, is controlled not by the battles you win or lose, with cancer or with anything else, but by the good you proclaim and imagine. In this sense, finally, are the crucifixion and resurrection stories of Jesus made most real; they constitute the poetic imaginations of the soul, not the prosaic rationalizations of earthly reason. One can never really see and name God in the world unless one first can imagine such a great goodness breaking into the world. It is only through such acts of imagination that one could possibly come to earth and begin by saying, "The Kingdom of God is at hand . . ."

What speaks to me most of that imaginative power is music. It is no accident that much of this book centers on metaphors of song and song lyrics. The combination of beautifully poetic words with richly evocative music provides me with my clearest intuitions of faith and Christian existence. In more than one religion, song is the gift of the gods; in C. S. Lewis's Narnia stories, song is the very voice of creation: the great Christ-figure, the terribly good Aslan, sings the world into existence. I find that to be so with me — worlds are created and recreated within my spirit via the agency of music. In one of the best appropriations and interpretations of the Arthurian theme in juvenile literature, Susan Cooper has created a young hero, Will, who plays out in the contemporary world the never-ending Arthurian struggle between good and evil. In what is, to me, one of the most fascinating episodes in the series, called "The Dark Is Rising," Will actually transforms reality by playing and singing Christmas music. That is paradigmatic for the way I think about the power of music.

The power of music. One composer in particular has power over me; his work lays bare the triumph of divinity as well as the delicateness of faith. His name is Ralph Vaughan Williams.

The triumph he portrays can be either bold or subtle. At the beginning of this chapter stands the first verse of "For All the Saints," a song for which Williams wrote the music. One of the most cherished moments of my life came when we stood for the final hymn at Melanie's funeral, a packed church energetically singing "For All the Saints." As the music swelled, I was caught up and enraptured — by the words, yes, but the music itself was a transport to heaven. As I stood there, singing a final song as the exclamation point to Melanie's life, a thrill ran through me; the hair stood up on the back of my neck. I felt pure triumph. The marvelous music coalesced with that glorious fifth verse:

> And when the fight is fierce, the warfare long,
> Steals on the ear the distant triumph song,
> And hearts are brave again, and arms are strong:
> Alleluia, Alleluia!

Melanie's life itself was part of the music of that distant triumph song, and through her living and dying the sound was brought closer, made clearer, rang louder. I don't think I have ever felt more Christian than at that moment in terms of the clarity of vision I had of the contours of the music of that distant land of pure Good News.

Of course, as I mentioned, not all moments are so clearly triumphant in Williams's music. Along with this bolder sense of triumph in "For All the Saints," there is another, subtler version of triumph found in his achingly beautiful "The Lark Ascending." If the music of "For All the Saints" represents those moments of rare, out-in-the-open, bold triumph that the Christian faith promises, the music of "Lark" is something altogether different, yet in many ways more sustaining. For it is music that, for me, is the tonal representation of my Christian faith as I live it out day by day. Although the piece is about a lark, I see the bird as a metaphor for the soul and its ascent to its proper sphere. It is a delicate piece, seemingly fragile at points, not unlike Christian faith; it suggests the times of uncertainty and doubt, of despair, when the striving to ascend seems at best a far-off dream. For me, the piece evokes bittersweet longings, a pang, a desire for flight. It is a longing for flight that seems almost as good as the flight itself; it is something that feeds the efforts to ascend, up and up, not through space and time but through dimensions of relationship, until one is finally, at the peak of the ascent, put into right relationship with the proper object of all desires, God.

The best analogy to this in strictly theological terms is, I believe, John Calvin's view of the Eucharist, when that view is adjusted a bit. Calvin thought that in the act of the Eucharist one was, by the power of the Holy Spirit, elevated to heaven, where one feasted on Christ and thereby obtained his benefits of forgiveness and eternal life. That is a Eucharistic language of ascent. Calvin thought of heaven as a place; if instead we think of heaven in relational rather than spatial terms, we get at what I think is going on both in Williams's "Lark" and in Calvin's teaching. The power of the music, just like the elements of the Eucharist, serves as an instrument that lifts the heart and soul into God's kingdom, understood not as a throne room above the skies but as a recognition that in our longings for the Good we are set on the path of ascent that puts us into a relationship of absolute trust in that Good — a Good that, through all the shadows of longing in earthly existence, finally raises us up to itself so that we might delight in it.

This may sound hopelessly romantic. But it is a romanticism that keeps me out of the pit of despair; it is the rope ladder that I ascend out of the pit into the light. That's the best of faith, and if I can't put it into words that are adequate, I can hear it in the music and taste it in the Eucharist. I would argue that just as Williams's "Lark" is romantic, so is the spirit of Christianity that it represents for me. Christian faith *is* romantic, at least in the sense of evoking these bittersweet longings, longings that represent to us the Absolute Good we desire, the thing that we are able to receive until that day when our spirits are in such a state as to be able to move beyond the longing to that which is longed for itself.

Again, does all of this make sense? Perhaps not. The best way I can put it is to say that, theologically, God is all powerful because even his absence produces joy. It is a somber, real joy, a longing that is, above all, a sweetness because of its very ability to communicate to us the need for that which is absent, and the promise that one day that which is hidden will be made bright as day, the day we no longer have to look through the dark mirror of longing to catch a glimpse of Pure Delight. Again, this may not make sense, but, of course, Melanie's dying makes no sense to me, either. And so, if the tragedy of death is finally a mystery that is inexplicable, may we have the good sense to accept the mystery of joy as well.

As I have thought through these issues, what has happened to me — something that is probably clear to those of you who know the writings of C. S. Lewis — is that I have come to an existential knowledge of what Lewis was talking about when he wrote about joy. He is the one who so well described joy as that which must have the stab, the pang, the inconsolable longing; he also talked about how all the small joys of life serve as a reflection of that great joy toward which all creation strives; the soul's journey to ultimate joy, God, is mapped out with these smaller markers of joy.

In that sense, again, Melanie serves as a mirror of joy for me. When I think of her now, I think of the beauty, grace, and goodness that she was. The sweet pang of longing, the joy, that I have for her resonates now with my piety. Joy itself, the feeling of longing after the good, is palpable in my existence now. It had been there before in small ways, but now . . . well. More than once I have thought for a long while about Melanie, and then the joy of having known her and the joy of longing have become so real that they have gripped my heart — I have audibly gasped at times, I have been so taken by the joy she represents. And if sometimes I look at our children and see my inadequacies as a parent, more and more I look and see joy. I see my friends who are so gracious to me, family members who help me out, and there is joy. Joy in the sense of a longing for the final consummation of Goodness, when it will no longer be in things external to me, such as mirrors and reminders, but will be written indelibly, deeply into my heart. I don't think it is twisting Saint Augustine too badly to say that this may capture at least part of what he meant when he asked of God, "How shall my heart rest, 'til it rest in Thee?" Joy as longing for the good is a path we travel until the day of rest, when Joy itself, as it really is, serves as home and haven.

We are all of us, then, travelers along the path, wayworn at times, yet often refreshed by the springs of joy. Travelers. In my church one Sunday, when people were offering prayer concerns, someone asked for traveling grace — that is, they were going on a trip and wanted prayers for their safe return. The minister misunderstood exactly how the request had been phrased; the result was that he said, "And we pray this morning for Grace, who's traveling." And while that at first struck me as a funny transposition, I thought about it and decided that it is true. The grace of God is no static thing, but it travels; it travels because of who we are in our journeys, and it is the thing which enables our journeys. Because we are all travelers, all the prayers we say are for traveling grace — that is, for a grace that accompanies us on our climbs up the sides of earthly existence. In that sense, there were no unanswered prayers during Melanie's illness; she was not cured, but she always had grace for the journey.

Where am I in my journey now, and how do I understand it? Or, to change the metaphor to the one I used at the beginning of the book, How do I sing the Lord's song? Often I experience my life as a single note, though perhaps God counts that as a song, or at least the beginning of a song. Sometimes I am the fragile violin lead in "The Lark Ascending"; at other times I see myself as part of the orchestral support for the motion of Melanie's soul as it took flight toward heaven. In her last sermon, Melanie herself talked of the music she heard, speaking of the love of God in Christ, a reckless love. She heard a music that she described as something that invited you to "suck in God's grace like invigorating mountain air." Mountain trail songs — that's what I sing on my own way up the mountain. And Melanie helped to teach me the tune; she is the Lark I follow and sing after.

I am able to sing because Melanie enabled me to sing, and through her memory she enables me to sing still. Melanie was and is a saint of God, a saint in Frederick Buechner's sense of the word: someone who makes you feel more alive. And it is in the painful joy of longing I now feel, in the moments I am faithful, that I am most alive to the possibility of the goodness of life. I wouldn't trade the pain of that joy for all the pleasures of life, because it is the surest indicator for me of the good that lies ahead, when God will be "all in all."

The melody of joyful longing was made clear to me in

quite a serendipitous event. I was cleaning out my desk one day when I came upon some old cassettes. My first impulse was to toss them, but I decided to play them first. And the first one I played was a tape of Melanie and me singing together sixteen years ago. I had completely forgotten the event and the song. But as soon as I heard the tape, everything came back to me. Melanie and I had been practicing a song for an outdoor worship service at a state park, a service we led when we were in college. In my mind's eye I could still see the dress Melanie had worn that day. We had practiced the song over and over again on the tape in order to improve our rendition of it. I wept as I heard us singing together. The words were simple: "Think about things that are pure and loving, / think about things that are good and true. / Dwell on the finer things in others, / think about all that God can do. / And be glad about it, / and sing for Joy, / And be glad about it, / and sing to the Lord." Now I sing this song to my children at night, every night. In its simple language, it says all that needs to be said: goodness, truth, Joy, gladness, and God are all tied together by our songs in praise to God, whether they be the songs of our lips, our hearts, or our lives. And because all of that is focused for me by a song — which is, it turns out, the only recording I have of Melanie and me singing together — it also focuses my longing for Melanie in a good way that points toward all that is fine in this world, and all that will be finer in the next.

John Calvin, through a catechism he wrote, taught children that the chief end of human existence is to glorify God and enjoy him forever. It used to be that when I read that line I made the mistake of thinking that the chief end was composed of two things: glorifying and enjoying. But I now realize that the two are one. The glory is the enjoyment. In other words, to recognize and name God's glory (his goodness, his desirability, his love) even when a loved one dies — indeed, even when one is in the midst of the loved one's dying — is to be placed within Joy itself (en-joy-ment).

> Sing, ye heights of heav'n, his praises;
> angels and archangels, sing!
> Wheresoe'er ye be, ye faithful,
> let your joyous anthems ring,
> ev'ry tongue his name confessing,
> countless voices answering,
> evermore and evermore!

So goes the last verse of "Of the Father's Heart Begotten." Because of the joy I associate with Melanie now, I am open, in my better moments, to the countless voices that sing God's praises and thus enjoy his presence. And as long as I can hear the countless voices, however dim, however distant, I can echo the song. And this is, in the end, the final lesson I have learned: wherever the music of joy is heard — that longing, bittersweet, delicate sound, the tonal vision of the Lark that finally ascends to the heavens — there are no strange lands; they all are footpaths to God.

EPILOGUE

A Better Country

> *Like cold water to a thirsty soul,*
> *so is good news from a far country.*
>
> — Proverbs 25:25

> *These all died in faith, not having received what was promised, but having seen it and greeted it from afar. . . . As it is, they desire a better country, that is, a heavenly one.*
>
> — Hebrews 11:13a, 16a

This epilogue is, for the most part, a fairy story, but I should explain its genesis. Two things are involved.

Predictably, Mave and Gwynne ask me where Mommy is. When I answer "Heaven," they ask the inevitable question: "Where is heaven?" As Mave points out, when you go up in a rocket ship, it's not there. The best explanation I can give, particularly because I believe that heaven has less to do with space (except metaphorically) than with a relationship, is this: "Heaven is the place we call God's heart. Just as Mommy is in your heart, so Mommy is in God's heart, and that's heaven." I stop there with them, but I go on to myself: The difference is that Mommy in our hearts is a memory of something gone, whereas Mommy in God's heart is made alive by God's holy memory, where words and reality do not suffer the chasm of disconnection they do in human life.

The notion of Mommy in heaven ties into another wish that the children have strongly expressed: When they die, they want to go to heaven and be the same age they were when Mommy died, with Mommy, of course, being the same age she was when she died. In other words, they wish that heaven will be a place where life, real life, can pick up where it left off.

There are other purple flower fairy stories in this book: the previous ones were written by Melanie. The one that follows here is one I wrote, partly to provide a good ending to the purple flower fairy stories, and partly to address the two concerns Mave and Gwynne have.

In this story I've switched the name of the little girl from Mave to Layne. Up until now, Mave has been the name of the little girl in the purple flower fairy stories — which stands to reason, because Melanie wrote them for Mave, just as she wrote other stories for Gwynne. For the purposes of this book, I've used mainly the purple flower fairy stories. This doesn't mean that the stories Melanie wrote for Gwynne aren't important; they just aren't as clearly evocative of the sorts of things I want to say as the fairy stories are. Still, since this is a new story I've written, and because I've written it in response to the needs and questions of both my children, the story is, in a sense, about both of them — and that's why I've used the name "Layne." "Layne" is a variant of "Lane," which was Melanie's last name and is both Mave and Gwynne's middle name. So "Layne" is a singular name for Mave and Gwynne together. I've also changed the purple flower fairy from a she to a he. In providing a conclusion for Melanie's stories, I've written a story that is also clearly my own.

In this story I use the metaphor of space to try to say something about God's heart. On the one hand, the story is the most obviously fictional thing I've written in this book; on the other hand, if this book really is to mean anything at all, the story has to be the truest thing I've written.

The Purple Flower Fairy Flies Layne Home

Years passed. Layne began to wonder if the purple flower fairy was ever really real. She grew up. She became old. But always, by her bedside, she kept the last purple flower the fairy had given her. It had to be real, Layne would think. But, then again, maybe it was just all her imagination.

One night, there was a glow in Layne's room. She woke up, and there he was! The purple flower fairy.

"Oh!" Layne cried. "You're back! I'm so glad you're back. I knew you'd come back." Tears formed in her eyes.

"Yes, I'm back," said the fairy. "And I've come for you. Walk to me, Layne."

Layne jumped out of bed. She was so happy! But then she noticed something, something she had not noticed before. The purple flower fairy was not purple — he was white. And she found it to be almost a blinding kind of white when she tried to look directly at him. He seemed to be different. In the blurry white he seemed to change forms — sometimes he looked like a beautiful white lily, sometimes a gorgeous white rose. He was majestic in his beauty, grand in his whiteness.

"You've changed," Layne offered. Not in a judgmental tone or a surprised tone. She was just stating a fact.

"No, Layne, dear one. You have changed. But it's for the better. You'll see." And the fairy laughed a long, deep laugh, one that bubbled over, almost visible in its joyfulness. "Look behind you, Layne."

Layne turned and looked. The first thing she saw was surprising enough. She had wings. Not the sort of temporary wings the purple flower fairy had always given her before, but big, lovely, intricate wings, with the shape of hearts interwoven in their design. But then Layne saw something else that quite made her forget about her wings.

Layne saw herself lying on the bed — peaceful, restful looking. She walked over, bent over herself on the bed, and touched the figure who lay there.

"Am I, am I, what . . ." Layne stammered.

"Yes, Layne, you have died, dear heart. But, in dying, you are now more alive than you have ever been before. Come! Come fly with me! I will take you to a special place where only the wings you have now can take you. Run, and jump, and fly!" With that, the purple flower fairy (for that is how Layne still thought of him, despite his change of colors) glided out the window.

Layne went out after him. Once outside, she tumbled in the air, straightened out, and flew upward, upward, ever upward. Higher and higher she flew. Lands, planets, and solar systems seemed to fly past her. Then she experienced an odd sensation. She continued to fly, but she no longer seemed to be moving. She seemed to be stationary in the air, like a hummingbird, while things around her simply grew blurry and then seemed to disappear — not because of distance; it was a different kind of change. Then blurry images began to appear again, but they were different from the ones before. She was traveling; she knew that. But it was no longer through "places." It was a different kind of traveling. Soon the fuzzy images took on sharpness, a sharpness that Layne was sure would cut her to shreds; she had never seen images so bright, so real, so full. There emerged all around her a land of indescribable beauty, a land of gigantic dimensions. Yet the beauty of the things she saw surpassed even their size. Finally, she seemed to see that there was a center to the wondrous land: a tremendously large waterfall. It looked to be hundreds, maybe thousands, of miles away, yet she could make out every drop of mist that rose from the base of the falls. It had to be, she thought, the largest thing in the whole universe; certainly it was bigger than the galaxies she had passed on her way to this land. Yet, despite its great size, she could take it all in. And she thought that the beauty that radiated from it, the light that shone off its every little drop of water, was the beauty that was cast over the entire land.

"Where are we?" Layne asked the purple flower fairy.

The purple flower fairy looked kindly on Layne and replied, "Layne, dear, we are in God's heart. It's a place that, back in your other world, you dimly imagined as heaven."

"It's so big!" Layne exclaimed.

"Oh yes," the purple flower fairy laughed. "Big indeed. But not in the way you are used to thinking about big. This place is so big that for all of eternity you can fly around and never see the end of it. But it can also fit inside the heart of a small child. Yes," the purple flower fairy said, "it is big, the biggest thing there is. But it's the sort of thing that has nothing to do with size."

Layne pondered the fairy's words for a few minutes. It was during this time that she became aware of a sound. She could never tell after that if she hadn't been aware of it at first because it was too loud or too soft. But eventually her ears became attuned to the noise, and the noise was laughter. Once she heard it, she realized that it was everywhere: above her, below her, ahead of her, behind her. It seemed to ripple through the air, shake the ground, run along across the top of the waters, sing through the trees. It was everywhere.

The laughter was the most joyous sound Layne had ever heard. And though it was everywhere, she realized that there was a source from which it sprang: the waterfall, those crystal falls that shone beauty. As she looked more carefully at the falls, she saw a strange thing: at the base of the falls, the water that had fallen from such an incredibly high distance was gathered and shot back up through the air — it was less like an earthly waterfall basin, Layne thought, and more like a fountain. And all of a sudden she knew that that fountain, where the roar of the falling water should have been loudest, was where the laughter was springing from. And then she knew: that fountain of goodness was the center of God's heart. And she also knew something else: the laughter that ran out from that place did not ripple the air — it *was* the air, the very air that she breathed, the air that supported her wings in flight.

Layne turned to the purple flower fairy. "Who is that?" she asked, pointing to the waterfall. She knew it wasn't a what; it had to be a who, for only a "who" could make such delicious laughter. The fairy said, "That is my Father, and I must now go to him." And as he said that, he laughed with a laughter Layne now recognized as a sound just like the one she heard coming from the falls.

"But if you go, who will stay with me?" Layne inquired.

"Don't worry about that," the purple flower fairy replied. "Your guide is coming now. Good-bye, dear heart. We shall meet again before long." And with those words, the fairy was off to that far-distant waterfall, at a speed of incomprehensible swiftness, so that within seconds he was at the basin of the falls, at the fountain, and then, in the next instant, he disappeared into the mist. At that same moment, Layne saw what she thought looked like a bird of some kind — a dove, perhaps — of the same brilliant whiteness as the fairy and the falls, dive into the mist from above. At that moment, the laughter in the air did not change — but it did seem to Layne that it was about three times louder.

Layne now turned her attention to her guide, coming ever closer. All of a sudden, Layne recognized the figure: it was Mommy! Mommy was coming to her, and it was the same Mommy she remembered from her childhood, a Mommy young and strong and beautiful, with flowing brown hair surrounding her like a halo. Layne then noticed herself; she was no longer an old woman but a seven-year-old child.

The reunion was gladness itself. As laughter surrounded them, Mommy looked at Layne and smiled a smile of Real Joy, a smile that threw in relief the shadowland joy of earth; a smile that shattered the boundaries of hope and longing, as that which Layne had so long hoped for was replaced by the real thing. Mommy held Lane with a look of love and said, "This is a better country, Layne. And the further you go in, the better it is. Come, dear little one, let's go together." And so, hand in hand, Layne and Mommy flew off to explore the country of Pure Joy.